Strategies for behavioral issues and **practical tips** for caring for your loved one at home

Dementia
for Caregivers

The complete guide for caregivers and families with explanations of *7 types of dementia*

RENEE PHILLIPPI

DEMENTIA FOR CAREGIVERS

STRATEGIES FOR BEHAVIORAL ISSUES AND
PRACTICAL TIPS FOR CARING FOR YOUR LOVED ONE
AT HOME – THE COMPLETE GUIDE FOR CAREGIVERS
AND FAMILIES WITH EXPLANATIONS OF 7 TYPES OF
DEMENTIA

RENEE PHILLIPPI

CONTENTS

Part III
YOU AND YOUR FUTURE

INTRODUCTION

Maybe you've found yourself in this position with little warning. You're doing the best you can for your loved one. You're drained, exhausted, and overwhelmed. You may not have any other option other than to continue on as the primary caregiver.

According to the World Health Organization, roughly 55 million people are affected by a form of dementia, and this number is expected to double by 2050 (World Health Organization, 2021). Despite Alzheimer's being, by far, the most common form of dementia, saying that the two terms are equal would be incredibly wrong. In fact, dementia is only an umbrella term, including different conditions – such as Lewy Body, Vascular Dementia, and many more.

Any person affected by dementia will likely need some form of caregiving. During the early stages, caregiving can be sporadic and merely supportive. In the more advanced stages, a patient will need a full-time caregiver, offering help to support their motor, psychological, cognitive, and other difficulties. This situation is very impactful for caregivers who, in the US alone, provided around 16 billion hours of unpaid care in 2021 (Alzheimer's Association, 2022). Why unpaid? You might wonder. Because the great majority of them are family members. Most of the time, they are women taking care of their parents or spouses affected by dementia.

Most people talk about the pain of dementia patients, but the caregivers go through a lot too. As a caregiver, you constantly worry about your loved one and their needs. It's difficult to see them go through this disease and not be able to do anything about it. You constantly feel like you are running out of time and options, and it often seems like you're failing them. Long-term care options can be challenging to figure out emotionally and financially. Caring for someone with Dementia can also be very isolating. As your loved one's condition progresses, they may need more and more help with everyday tasks. This can make it hard to get out and socialize, which can also make you feel lonely.

As a caregiver, you are not alone in feeling frustrated and overwhelmed. According to the National Institute on Aging, more than 16 million Americans are caring for someone with Alzheimer's or other types of dementia. This number is expected to increase as the population ages. According to a National Family Caregivers Association study, approximately 65 percent of caregivers feel unprepared to care for their loved ones. Furthermore, 38 percent of caregivers report high-stress levels, and 34 percent say caregiving negatively impacts their health.

I was also one of those caregivers who felt like I was constantly treading water. I was juggling my career, my social life, and the never-ending financial stress of caring for a loved one with dementia. It wasn't easy finding a way to manage it all and still have a successful career, a social life, and low-stress levels, but then I realized that I wasn't alone. There are millions of other caregivers out there who are struggling just like me. So I decided to write a book about my experiences and how I overcame the challenges of caregiving. In it, I share my tips for managing stress, staying organized, and maintaining a positive outlook. I also talk about the importance of self-care and how to find support from others. By sharing my story, I hope to help other caregivers realize that they are not alone and that they can find success in caregiving just as I did.

My goal in writing this book was two-fold: First, our loved ones deserves for us to care for them in the very best way we can. Secondly, there needs to be more information available on how best we, as individuals, can help ourselves during these challenging times. Lack of information leaves most families feeling isolated and alone. This book is split into three convenient parts to provide an easy-to-understand guide for caregivers. I want to share the shortcuts I've learned so that you can feel confident and knowledgeable about dementia caregiving. This book will teach you what you need to know about dementia. From the basics of what it is and how it affects people to the best ways to care for someone with the condition. You'll learn about the different types of dementia and the symptoms they cause, as well as how the disease progresses. Most importantly, you'll get practical tips and advice on how to be a caring and effective caregiver for someone with dementia.

Caring for someone with dementia can be taxing, both emotionally and physically. This book is unique because it offers practical tips and advice from caregivers with first-hand experience with the condition. This resource is designed to help caregivers of all levels of experience. It doesn't matter if you've been caring for a loved one with dementia for years or if you are just starting this journey. This guide will give you the information and support needed to make the best decisions for yourself and your loved one. This book will also offer tips and advice on how to take care of yourself. You cannot pour from an empty cup.

PART I

UNDERSTANDING DEMENTIA

"There are only four kinds of people in the world. Those who have been caregivers. Those who are currently caregivers. Those who will be caregivers, and those who will need a caregiver."

— ROSALYN CARTER

1

TYPES AND CAUSES

Because this journey requires knowledge of the diseases you might have to confront as a caregiver, we'll learn what dementia is in this chapter. Included are highlights of seven forms of dementia and detailed information about each type. This is a pivotal part of the learning process because most confusion concerns the differentiation of conditions based on symptoms.

WHAT IS DEMENTIA?

Very generally speaking, dementia is a progressive decline of cognitive functions. Cognitive functions are mental processes that allow us to carry out any task. They include language, memory, problem-solving, and perception. They enable us to navigate the world around us.

When speaking about Alzheimer's in particular, semantic memory is the first type of memory loss that patients experience, even years before the diagnosis (Verma & Howard, 2012). This can manifest as difficulty in speaking and being verbally fluent but not hearing and understanding spoken words. Why so? You might wonder.

Imagine your brain as an oval container: it's made of roughly 86 billion neurons, which are cells that control every single part of you. When we say that dementia kills the cells in your brain, it means that, based on which region it attacks first, you will not be able to perform a specific action. Speaking and comprehending words, despite functioning as a shared network to enable communication, are controlled by different parts of your brain. This is why speaking difficulties should not be underestimated in older adults, just because their ability to understand is intact!

In the initial stages, dementia-related cognitive impairment might not be so visible and straightforward. There is a term that clinicians use to refer to a condition that lies between age-related decline and dementia: mild cognitive impairment or MCI. Individuals falling in this category show mild difficulties in tasks that require specific cognitive abilities, such as paying bills, shopping, or preparing food, but need no special assistance. There is a significant risk but no certainty that MCI will result in dementia. Still, it should also be noted that symptoms associated with MCI can be brought on by some medications and diseases and may be reversed.

According to the CDC, in 2014, the estimated number of adults with dementia was 5 million, with the expectation that number would reach 14 million by 2060.

Contrary to popular belief, dementia is not a part of normal aging. Some forgetfulness can be expected as one ages, like occasionally misplacing keys, forgetting a recent event, forgetting a friend's name, or struggling to find a word and later remembering it. However, many older adults never develop dementia.

7 TYPES OF DEMENTIA

Alzheimer's Disease

Alzheimer's Disease is the most common form of dementia, affecting roughly 6.5 million Americans aged 65 and older who are living with it in 2022. As of 2019, it was the sixth leading cause of death in the US (Alzheimer's and Dementia). It was first reported in 1906 by the German Clinical Psychiatrist and Neuroanatomist Alois Alzheimer, after whom the disease is named. In his report, he noted distinctive plaques and neurofibrillary tangles in the brain of a 50-year-old female patient that he'd had under his care and followed until the time of her death. She'd exhibited symptoms of memory loss, hallucinations, paranoia, and confusion until her death, just five years after her admission to his service. Alzheimer published three more cases in 1909 and an additional case in 1911 of a patient with plaques only. Alzheimer died of heart failure in 1915.

After years of research, we now know that Alzheimer's first impacts working memory (the ability to remember information kept in mind for a short time to perform cognitive tasks), but, in the long run, it also destroys other parts of the brain. As the disease progresses, other cognitive abilities can be affected, such as speaking, learning, making weighted judgments, and controlling mood and behaviors. This continues until the long-term memory and the capacity for movements are entirely disrupted. Thus, saying that Alzheimer's Disease involves memory loss is only partly true: it involves an irreversible cascade of cell death. The APO(E) gene has been identified as a gene that shows an increased risk of developing Alzheimer's. A blood test can be done to determine whether one has the gene. However, it does not mean the person with the gene will get the disease, just that there is an increased risk of developing it.

Some symptoms of Alzheimer's Disease are:

- Forgetting recently learned information,
- Forgetting events and appointments,
- Increased difficulty planning or organizing,
- Confusion about what day it is or where you are,
- Forgetting material you just read,

- Taking longer to do familiar tasks
- Having difficulty following a favorite recipe,
- Putting things in unusual places (milk in the pantry, keys in the refrigerator, dirty clothes in the trash instead of the hamper, etc.),
- Less attention to personal grooming

The part of the brain that affects learning is usually where Alzheimer's Disease first attacks, so friends and family may notice a change before the individual with symptoms does. A doctor should be consulted as soon as possible if you or your loved one suspects Alzheimer's.

In Alzheimer's, we see an abnormal accumulation (clumping) of plaques and tangles in the brain, usually starting in the hippocampus and spreading to other parts of the brain. Plaques are deposits of beta-amyloid, which is a protein that builds up in the spaces between nerve cells. Tangles are fibers of twisted proteins called tau. (pronounced like "wow"). Tangles build up inside cells. This clumping in the brain further causes neuronal (nerve cell) death, eventually leading to brain atrophy and shut-down. A cure for Alzheimer's disease has not been found yet, despite research being conducted for over 100 years.

Currently, the most used treatments are cholinesterase inhibitors. These medications increase the concentrations of acetylcholine in the brain, a fundamental neurotransmitter (a chemical messenger that allows communication between your brain cells), allowing memory formation, learning, muscle control, and other vital functions. In addition to the cholinesterase inhibitors, another medication often used is an NMDA (N-methyl-D-aspartate) receptor antagonist. This medication is sometimes used with or instead of cholinesterase inhibitors. However, very promisingly, there are currently several other vaccines under clinical trials as candidates to provide a cure for Alzheimer's. These vaccines intend to deplete the excess plaques and tangles in the brain (Precision Vaccination, 2022).

There are two drugs for Alzheimer's that were fast-tracked (accelerated approval) by the FDA and are controversial due to the side effects and interpretation of the study data results.

In June 2021, the FDA approved the use of Aducanumab, a monoclonal antibody, for the treatment of Alzheimer's disease. Biogen, the maker of Aducanumab, states that their drug reduces beta-amyloid by binding to and removing amyloid beta plaques. The estimated cost of this drug is around $28,000 per year. It's unclear how much, if any, of the cost Medicare and private insurers will cover for this drug.

Also, in June 2021, Bristol Myers Squibb purchased exclusive rights from biotechnology company Prothena for their new beta-amyloid-reducing drug. In October 2022, the FDA also approved the use of PRX005 by Prothena. Prothena says its monoclonal antibody can bind to and clear two types of plaques with about 11 times more strength than Aducanumab. In clinical trials, reduction of the beta-amyloid plaques showed a reduction in the decline of some patients with Alzheimer's Disease. Neither drug will restore lost memories. Ask your healthcare provider for more information.

Vascular Dementia

Vascular dementia is the second most common type of dementia, although less known than Alzheimer's. Like Alzheimer's, the likelihood of developing this dementia increases with age, accounting for 20% of dementia cases in the United States (Wolters & Ikram, 2019). In contrast with Alzheimer's, there are a variety of different causes behind this disease. The most common cause is hemodynamic disorder, where the normal blood supply to the brain is interrupted due to a blockage, which is known as a stroke. Other causes can be hemorrhages, blood vessel narrowing, and thromboembolisms, where small clots from arteries impair normal blood flow. Due to the similar symptoms shared with Alzheimer's, in the 20th century, there was still a significant overlap between the two. In 1974 Canadian neuroscientist Vladimir Hachinski described this form as "multi-infarct dementia," separating it from all the other forms. Multi-infarct dementia and vascular dementia are the same. However, one of the most significant indicators of vascular dementia, if no brain scans are performed, is the manner in which the symptoms worsen. This disease usually exhibits a stepwise decay, meaning that an individual can experience an abrupt deterioration in a given cognitive function after a stroke but then be steady and stable until the following one (Masson, 2022).

Progression of Alzheimer's disease

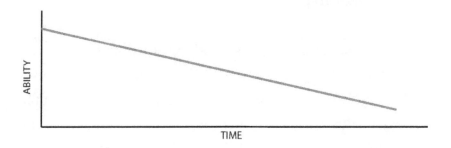

Progression of vascular dementia

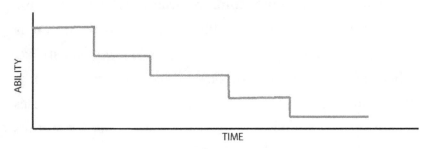

Difference of disease progression between Alzheimer's and vascular dementia.

Furthermore, Hachinski developed a scale to identify symptoms that can be specifically attributed to Vascular Dementia. These are specific neurological conditions such as limb paralysis, weakness, unusual reflexes, and severe depression. Specific to this type, after having one stroke, it's more likely that the person will have more, so it's essential to monitor the blood pressure and other indicators constantly. Like all the other forms of dementia, there is currently no cure. Because there are many causes, however, some things can be done to control the disease and make the life of the person affected more manageable. Maintaining a healthy diet is vital to reducing cholesterol, controlling diabetes, and managing high blood pressure, all of which reduce risk factors for vascular dementia. Subsequently, other things that can be done are quitting smoking and maintaining a healthy weight.

Lewy Body Dementia (LBD)

Lewy Body Dementia is named for Friedrick Lewy, a German neurologist who, in 1912, discovered abnormal protein deposits in people with Parkinson's Disease. (Coincidentally, Friedrick Lewy worked in the same lab as Alois Alzheimer). More than 1 million Americans are affected by Lewy body dementia. It has long been associated and confused with Alzheimer's due to the similarity of the underlying brain mechanisms. This disease also has a similar onset (50-85 years old) and tends to last four to four and a half years, although it has a maximal time range of one to twenty years. Like Alzheimer's, it's caused by an accumulation of proteins in the brain. Still, the symptoms, especially the initial ones, are quite different. In the early stages of the disease, patients usually experience visual hallucinations, states of confusion, and spatial disorientation. They can also experience muscular rigidity and tremors, symptoms of Parkinson's disease, which is a significant risk factor for LBD.

In contrast with Alzheimer's, the onset is also quite abrupt. The changes manifest more quickly, and memory is usually left intact. It took so long to differentiate the two conditions and give a singular identity to LBD because initial brain screening methods could not identify the Lewy bodies (which appeared as white) in the white matter of the brain (subcortical area containing nerve fibers). Only after the development of more sophisticated techniques could scientists identify those protein build-ups as being substantial enough to create brain damage. Like all the other forms of dementia, this one doesn't have a cure. Because Lewy Body disease is also characterized by a lack of acetylcholine in the brain, drugs used to treat Alzheimer's are also beneficial. Patients usually live around five to eight years after the onset of obvious LBD symptoms. Still, they can also live up to 20 years (Fernandes, 2010).

It should also be noted that Lewy body dementia is an umbrella term for two related diagnoses. The first related diagnosis is dementia with Lewy bodies. Individuals who develop Dementia with Lewy Body symptoms may also have a slight tremor and other changes in movement related to Parkinsonism. Not to get too far in the weeds here, but

Parkinsonism is a term that describes some neurological disorders similar to Parkinson's disease. The other form of LBD will also present with changes in movement. It may eventually be diagnosed as Parkinson's disease dementia.

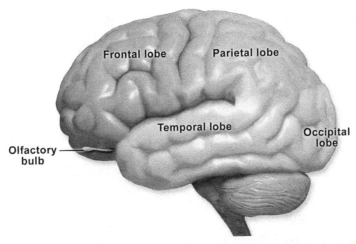

Depiction of the brain showing its lobes each having different functions

Parkinson's Disease

Parkinson's disease is a neurodegenerative condition and a form of dementia affecting nearly one million people in the US (Parkinson's Foundation, 2019). According to the Parkinson's Foundation, more than 10 million worldwide are living with PD. Men are 1.5 times more likely to have this disease than women. This disease was first medically described by the English surgeon James Parkinson, who published a breakthrough essay (An Essay on Shaking Palsy) describing it in 1817 (Parkinson, 1969). The condition was later named Parkinson's disease by Jean-Martin Charcot in honor of the English surgeon. Because the primary brain region this disease affects is the substantia nigra (forming part of the basal ganglia), patients develop severe difficulties with body movements. This is because when the substantia nigra is disrupted, its ability to produce dopamine is also impaired. Dopamine is a crucial neurotransmitter that regulates important body functions, among which movement is a key feature. All patients affected by this disease will experience tremors, limb stiffness, disrupted coordination, and difficulties with initiating movements overall. The causes underlying these diseases are still unknown. Still, some of the most accounted for are genetic and environmental factors, aging, and oxidation. A cure for Parkinson's hasn't yet been discovered, but two of the most widely used drugs used to treat its symptoms are Carbidopa and Levodopa, which spur the creation of new dopamine by crossing the blood-brain barrier. Since 1996, another highly effective treatment for essential tremors and severe tremors in PD patients has been Deep Brain Stimulation (DBS).

Frontotemporal Dementia

Frontotemporal dementia can also be considered an umbrella term to describe different types of conditions affecting the frontal and temporal lobes of the brain. It accounts for 1.7 to 7% of all dementia cases. (Leroy et al.,

2021). It's different from Alzheimer's in a variety of different ways. Firstof all, it has an earlier onset. The disease can arise starting from 35 years of age until 75, making it a common condition among the younger population. Second, the brain areas affected are different from Alzheimer's. This type of dementia primarily affects the frontal lobes (located in the front part of your brain, right underneath the forehead). It affects the capacity for judgement and reasoning, causing behavioral changes such as socially inappropriate behavior, aggressiveness, and general apathy. It also affects the temporal lobes of the brain (found deep down in the cerebral structure, behind the ears), which compromises speech abilities. Patients suffering from the latter usually have difficulties finding words and remembering people's names. The disease will progress into the loss of fluent speech. A key difference between Frontotemporal and Alzheimer's dementia is that the first doesn't usually involve memory loss, as the brain areas affected are different. However, similar to Alzheimer's, this dementia is characterized by the formation of plaques and tangles, which will eventually cause an excessive build-up and cell death. Unfortunately, there is currently no treatment that can reverse the course of this disease, and the medications usually prescribed are anti-depressants and antipsychotics, which help manage its symptoms.

Early-Onset Dementia

Younger or early-onset dementia refers to all the abovementioned subtypes but occurs in individuals younger than 65. Worldwide, approximately 3.9 million people under 65 may be affected. As we have seen, dementia can come as early as 35 years of age, like the frontotemporal case, and disrupt individuals' lives in different ways. Because dementia is an umbrella term, in this case, symptoms are multiple. A young patient can experience memory loss, the ability to make resonated judgments and perform simple tasks, as well as changes in their behaviors, attention, concentration, and social skills. It's hard and time-consuming to diagnose due to patients and physicians attributing many of the symptoms to stress, depression, or anxiety. Overall, Alzheimer's disease is the most common cause of young-onset dementia. Still, for those who develop symptoms before age 50, vascular and frontotemporal dementia are more likely the cause. Dr. David S. Knopman, a neurologist at the Mayo Clinic in Rochester, MN pointed out in a JAMA editorial in July of 2021 that many individuals diagnosed with young onset dementia are often in their 40s and 50s, may be raising children and are usually not ready to retire.

Chronic Traumatic Encephalopathy (CTE)

This type of dementia is developed following multiple traumatic brain injuries, which are ways through which your brain can be disrupted if the head receives strong blows. Rather than being a specific type of dementia, it refers to the general symptoms that an individual exhibits before developing a specific type of dementia. Symptoms include cognitive decline (memory loss, attentional difficulties, disorientation, and confusion), mood changes, Parkinsonism, speech impairment, and so on. Due to its nature, this disease is usually associated with contact sports, such as boxing, football, martial arts in general, or any sport that would cause repetitive blows over the years. Recent studies have suggested that the neuropathology of this condition can manifest through plaques and tangles similar to Alzheimer's and medial-temporal lobe atrophy (Baugh et al., 2014), triggering the cerebral disruptions we have discussed above. Treatments are still being developed, and there are currently different promising candidates. For example, immunotherapy to target tangles accumulation is one of the most studied techniques, as well as anti-inflammation techniques to contract the danger of neuroinflammation caused by brain injuries decreasing the protective role of certain molecules (Breen & Krishnan, 2020).

2

BRAIN PHYSIOLOGY AND ITS PROGRESSION

This chapter will provide a comprehensive picture of the physiological changes occurring in a dementia-affected brain. It will also walk you through the different stages in which the condition can manifest. This explanation will help you understand the severity of brain changes and prepare you to pinpoint specific symptoms of disease progression. While similar brain mechanisms trigger most dementia subtypes, we will focus on Alzheimer's hallmarks. By the end of this chapter, you'll have learned what occurs in the brain of your patients and what contributed to making their condition so impairing.

KEY BIOLOGICAL MECHANISMS OF THE HEALTHY BRAIN

Before diving into what occurs in a dementia-affected brain, it's fundamental for you to learn or re-learn some vital biological mechanisms that make all brains function correctly regarding communication, metabolism, repair, and regeneration. We have already said that the disruption of neuron communication causes cell death, but what is neuron communication in the first place, and why is it so fundamental for our survival?

Communication

Neurons, your brain cells, are the smallest units of your nervous tissue. Thanks to their communication, humans can perform cognitive, motor, and behavioral tasks. To have an idea of what a neuron looks like, consider the branch-like structure on the left in the image below. The image magnification shows the moment when two neurons exchange information. This happens rapidly (roughly 0.5 milliseconds) to allow individuals to perform every single task. Our thoughts, motor actions, intentions, memory, feelings, and emotion, are all dictated by neural communication.

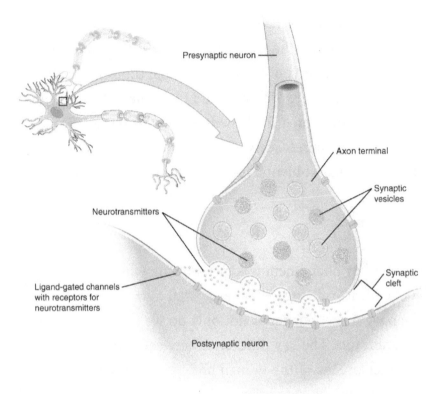

Depiction of a Neuron

When the latter is disrupted, as we'll see in the following paragraphs, all our abilities to perform even the simplest tasks are compromised too.

To have an idea of how complex and magnificent this whole system is, think about what happens in your brain all the time. Every single neuron is able to connect with 10,000 other neurons passing and receiving information through the help of one quadrillion synapses! (Zhang, 2019). A synapse is a fundamental agent for neural communication. It is the bubble-like yellow portion (pictured) that sends signals from one neuron to the others. These signals are also called neurotransmitters (the little green dots in the picture), and this is a word that you will read multiple times in this book. This is because many different and fundamental neurotransmitters are disrupted in dementia-affected brains. Some of these are dopamine, acetylcholine, and serotonin. They all serve different but pivotal functions for human survival.

Metabolism

Another key phenomenon is metabolism, which refers to the biochemical exchange of energy that our brain feeds on. When we ingest nutrients, not only do we feed our body but our brain too! The key difference between our brain and all the other organs of the human body is that it's able to draw its energy supply from only one nutrient: glucose. Glucose is a simple sugar that is contained in the majority of foods we intake. Fruit, vegetables, meat, cereals, cheese, and herbs all have a percentage of glucose, on which our brain is able to feed and draw the energies it needs to function. However, because it is not able to store glucose for an extended period of time (in contrast with the lipid supplies that our body stores as a survival strategy), it constantly needs an intake of glucose and oxygen from the blood. This is the reason why even a brief oxygen and glycemic drop might severely compromise the functioning of your brain. Another interesting consideration is the amount of energy expenditure our brain consumes when thinking about how small of an organ it is compared to others in our body. It consumes as much as 60% of glucose intake and 20% of oxygen while only making up 2% of the overall body mass! (Camandola & Mattson, 2017). However, as hard to believe as it might be, your brain's energy expenditure does not change much depending on the tasks you are performing. Whether you're sleeping or engaging in a cognitively demanding task, the blood influx to that organ doesn't change. It will always receive about a seventh of the overall cardiac output (blood coming from the heart), which is a lot if considering the brain size. As you might imagine, changes in these metabolic functions, if severe enough, might lead to physiological imbalances for which your body cannot carry out essential survival tasks. As we will see, dementia severely impacts your brain's capacity to carry out metabolic tasks, putting patients' lives increasingly in danger every day.

Repair, Remodelling, and Regeneration

The word regeneration related to your body might remind you of scar healing, hair growth, or anything that can be repaired. Even without an injury or lesion, most of your cells are constantly renewed because they undergo a life cycle, like every living organism. While most of the human system regenerates, neurons don't, apart from a few exceptions. This makes your brain an extremely vulnerable organ because its neurons live in a very challenging and hostile environment. If you go back to the neuron picture, you will notice that the axon is the longest arm of a brain cell. Suppose any section of the axon is damaged, the neurons can't communicate properly.

Furthermore, the myelin sheath (a fatty protective covering on axons that allows fast communication) around surrounding axons and astrocytes are protective agents which, as part of their jobs, prevent new axons from re-growing to avoid damaging the living ones. Despite the inability of the brain to re-grow its cells, it is equipped with another function to make up for the lost tissue: have you ever heard of the expression "brain plasticity"? If the dead neurons cannot re-grow, then the living ones will upgrade. Living neurons understand when they have a dead neighbor to which they can't connect and will establish new connections with other neurons to perform similar tasks! Because plasticity depends on surviving cells, the fewer the remaining cells, the less likely an individual will re-learn to do something. This is the reason why severe strokes, head injuries, and late stages of dementia can impact the life of someone so extensively.

DEMENTIA BRAIN

Amyloid Plaques and Neurofibrillary Tangles

We have said that dementia is neurodegenerative, meaning that it progressively causes the death of neurons. We have also mentioned the terms tangles and plaques multiple times, which affect neural communication. Let us see how. Alzheimer's disease develops when misfolded proteins cluster inside and outside of neurons. One of these proteins is called amyloid-beta, which is typically found in the extra-cellular space around neurons. In healthy brains, this protein is important for neuroprotection, as well as synaptic signalling and elasticity, promoting learning and memory. In Alzheimer's brains, however, these proteins clump together, forming one of the hallmarks of the disease: amyloid plaques. Another characteristic of this disease is the misfolding of a protein called tau, which in healthy brains is fundamental for maintaining the neural structure of micro-tubules. Microtubules make up the cell's skeletons.

As you can see in the picture below, the misfolding of tau protein also causes the disintegration and accumulation of tau protein tangles within the cell structure itself. In this way, the neuron lacking its internal structure is not able to send and receive signals anymore. This combination of events ultimately disrupts neural communication, eventually causing brain atrophy and cell death.

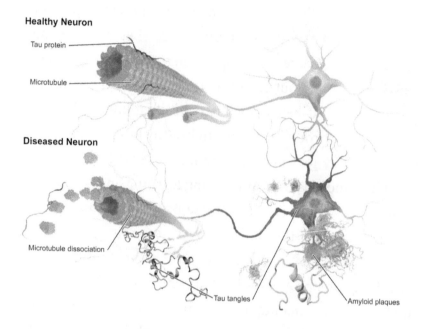

Healthy Neuron

Tau protein ——————

Microtubule ——————

Diseased Neuron

Microtubule dissociation

Tau tangles

Amyloid plaques

Healthy and Diseased Neurons Compared

THE SEVEN STAGES OF DEMENTIA

We have extensively mentioned that all types of dementia are progressive, meaning that very rarely will a patient exhibit an abrupt cognitive decline from one day to another. Instead, the disease usually progresses in stages, which differentiate from one another based on symptoms. It's widely accepted that dementia can be divided into seven different stages, following the seven-stage model (Reinsberg et al., 1982). severe Alzheimer's disease.

Stage 1 - No Impairment

The very first stage is when no symptoms are visible, but the disease has already started its course in the brain. Cerebral degradation occurs long before the slightest memory slip is detectable. An example is tau tangles which, if detected by a brain scan, can help predict the location and future spatial distribution of brain atrophy a year before the first symptoms become visible. Amyloid PET scans, which can show signs of amyloid clumps up to two decades before symptoms (Bhandari, 2021), can be useful for diagnosing dementia before symptoms appear.

Stage 2 - Very Mild Cognitive Decline

Stage two could be referred to as "Slight Cognitive Decline" when the first signs of memory or cognitive confusion start to occur in a patient but might still go undetected. Because the patient's social and organizational skills are still intact, they pass unnoticed the majority of the time. Common symptoms of this stage are misplacing keys, forgetting familiar names, or the position of frequently used objects. These innocent memory slips can happen to anyone.

Stage 3 - Mild Cognitive Decline

During the third stage, mild cognitive declines start to catch people's attention. This is because the memory slips are related to recently occurring things or names learned. A patient in this stage might also start experiencing trouble finding the correct words or misusing words in ways never before. Working memory is usually the first skill to be impaired. Symptoms of this are the inability to consolidate new short-term memories: an individual might start having trouble remembering a name just heard, a passage read in a book, or a recent conversation. Concentration and attention are more difficult too, which might start affecting an individual's working life. Planning and organizational skills, similarly, require a more significant mental effort, and routine tasks (such as taking meds and going to an appointment) are usually forgotten more frequently. However, because the symptoms of this stage can exist for three or four years before progressing to the following stage, dementia is usually not yet diagnosed.

Stage 4 - Moderate Cognitive Decline (early-stage dementia)

Diagnosis most often occurs at stage four, where the cognitive impairments become entirely noticeable. All the symptoms mentioned above tend to worsen, while others add up visibly. For example, long-term memory slips start to occur, where the patient forgets - or at least needs more effort to remember - events from the far past, while social and behavioral aspects decline too. Symptoms of withdrawal, apathy, and irritability begin to impact the social life of a patient, who at the same time will exhibit denial and refusal to acknowledge their condition. Because the cognitive and behavioral skills are significantly worsening, the individual will start needing part-time care and support from their family.

Stage 5 - Moderately Severe Cognitive Decline (mid-stage dementia)

A patient enters stage five when they start needing a full-time caregiver because the cognitive decline is severe enough to impact their daily life. In practical terms, this means that episodes of confusion (both spatial and mental), feelings of being lost, and forgetting relatives' names are more frequent. Because long-term memory is not entirely compromised, a patient might still be able to remember information about their identity: who they are, their adolescence, relatives' faces, and generally their history. Nevertheless, cognitive difficulties might impair critical aspects of their daily life. A patient in this stage might need special assistance to prepare their meals, get dressed, or any cognitively demanding task will need to be looked after. On the other hand, tasks concerning the person's primal needs, such as using the toilet, might still be carried out by the patient alone.

Stage 6 - Severe Cognitive Decline (late mid-stage dementia)

Stage six is usually referred to as "middle dementia," where, along with the severe cognitive decline, the patient will experience even worse physical difficulties. At this stage, a caregiver will need to take complete care of the patient, who will need help with toileting and showering. Because the patient might still recall episodes of past life, this is a highly debilitating phase in which the person sadly acknowledges their condition and realizes the amount of care that they need. Due to this and to sleep pattern irregularities, the patient will also experience drastic mood changes, characterized mainly by agitation, anger, and depression. This phase can last up to three years, and their ability to speak undergoes worsening symptoms during this time.

Stage 7 - Very Severe Cognitive Decline (late-stage dementia)

The seventh and last stage of dementia is the hardest one to handle because the physiological capabilities of the patient start to surrender. Here, most individuals will have difficulty controlling their bowel movements and carrying out other tasks, such as swallowing and speaking. Speaking abilities might be almost completely lost, and the patient might not be able to articulate phrases. They may be able to say a few words, but they might be out of context and disconnected. Physical slowing might also impact walking and movements in general, given the dopamine deficiencies they will be experiencing. The difficulties in swallowing can cause recurrent pneumonia due to aspiration, which can put the patient's life at severe risk, given that their immune system is significantly compromised at this stage. However, if dementia is detected early enough, current treatments can slow down the progression of the disease and its symptoms.

WHAT DOES DEMENTIA FEEL LIKE?

Because we are slowly shifting from a broad medical perspective to an individual focus, we will soon address dementia, considering the patient's state of mind. As we have understood how dementia affects the brain, we should now discuss how this condition affects the patient. How do they notice the first warning signs of their cognitive decline? How do they deal with the heartbreaking news of their diagnosis? How do they adapt to their new life? We'll look at four stories from the perspective of the patient.

First, to really dive into the mind of a dementia-affected patient, it might be worth mentioning the award-winning movie "The Father." Before watching it, however, you should know that because it's so accurate, it might also be tough to watch and may be upsetting. If you choose to watch it, it may give you a deep insight into what it feels like to live with dementia. It speaks about a dementia-affected patient, played by Anthony Hopkins. His condition causes progressively more trouble in his perception of reality. While altering states of irritability and cheerfulness and refusing the care of his daughter, he slowly starts to look suspiciously at what his daughter and relatives do. This situation escalates until reaching very troubling states in his mind, leading him to question his whole existence and reality.

Katy Robinson, a 56-year-old outgoing and charming lady, first noticed something wrong with her when she couldn't find the words she was looking for during a conversation and, later, during a job presentation. She described this feeling as very confusing because she knew the word, but somehow she couldn't say it out loud. It's similar to the tip of the tongue state, where you know the word (the meaning, the context), but there is no way it will come out. She also started forgetting conversations or repeating things multiple times until her husband suggested going to see their doctor. Through a PET scan, she was diagnosed with posterior cortical atrophy, a subtype of Alzheimer's disease, specifically affecting spelling, calculating, and visual and spatial processing. She recalls hearing the diagnosis and feeling completely hopeless and desperate, expecting the worst consequences on her health and well-being. Thanks to the support of her husband and a few friends, things went better. She quit her job and became a member of the Alzheimer's Association's Early-Stage Advisory Group in order to take full care of herself.

Carla Benton, a Church Pastor and mother of three, was diagnosed with early-onset Alzheimer's disease at the age of 51. She, too, started noticing symptoms of general confusion and difficulties in finding the correct words. Still, she post-poned a medical check multiple times. This was due to her father having suffered from frontotemporal dementia, and the fear of being diagnosed with the same condition held her back. She also attributed her symptoms to the stress caused by the Covid-19 pandemic until she was faced with the truth. Her diagnosis was very debilitating for her. She didn't think there was truly something wrong with her, and it took her quite some time to acknowledge her situation. Being a pastor, she mostly relied on her faith and family support to first get familiar with her condition. She is now hopeful that her life won't change much for a long period of time, as she reports feeling happy, grateful for her life, and positive. She also applied to participate in a clinical trial at West Virginia University's Rockefeller Neuroscience Institute to access some medical treatments. She's hoping that they will work to slow the course of the disease and participating in a scien-tific study may help find a cure for all the other people affected by the disease.

Marc Jacobs, a 59-year-old procurement analyst, reports a more complex diagnostic history, for which it took him about three years to be diagnosed. His initial symptoms were slightly different from usual, resembling a form of dyslexia and dysgraphia (a neurological disorder that causes a person's writing to be distorted or incorrect) paired with general organizational difficulties. The initial doctor appointments didn't lead anywhere until he found more accurate words to describe his challenges. He told the doctor that he knew what a specific letter would look like, but he somehow forgot how to draw it. He also reported having difficulties choosing the right clothes and getting dressed, describing feelings of confusion and hopelessness. The day he finally got his posterior cortical atrophy diagnosis, he was also told he had to stop driving. From then on, his independence slowly decreased. After his experience, he advises anyone who feels insecure about themselves and their health to explain their symptoms to doctors with as much detail as possible. Feeling confused and uncertain is very common, and scientific advances are tailoring diagnostic problems every day to achieve better results.

Rick Landfield, a 72-year-old man, had a 30-year-long career in automotive manufacturing. Due to his job, he'd always been required to travel, taking trains and flights at least three times a week. Some of his first symptoms specifically affected his job because he frequently went to the wrong airports or train stations, and to appointments on the wrong days. At first, he attributed these errors to the stress of his busy work schedule and postponed a medical check for many years. At the age of 70, he had a stroke that severely impacted his working memory. His doctor ordered a PET scan, resulting in an Alzheimer's diagnosis. The worst thing about delaying the diagnosis is the loss of time to plan for the future. But, as he reported, it was also his point of strength. During most of his life, he was always forced to follow a rigid schedule. He now appreciates living in the moment, not caring too much about what will happen next.

These stories all witness the resilience and strong mindset of people who had to face the hard truth of being diagnosed with dementia. The diagnosis itself sometimes takes time, both because the symptoms don't show up right away as the brain health starts to deteriorate and because the risk of misdiagnosis is still very high. In the next chapter, we'll see how this process takes place, the importance of early diagnosis and its impacts on patients, and current treatment options.

3

THE DIAGNOSIS

For many years the diagnosis of dementia was mainly made through superficial screening, which did not deliver the most reliable results.

DIAGNOSING DEMENTIA

Pinpointing dementia (now also referred to as Major Neurocognitive Disorder) in a patient with memory problems is not so straightforward. While scientists and professionals acknowledge the limits of diagnostic criteria and work daily to develop new methods, they will still need to verify specific parameters to rule out other possible causes. Clinicians use a book called "The Diagnostic and Statistical Manual of Mental Disorders," better known as "DSM-5-TR". What is it, and why is it helpful? The first version of this manual was first written in 1952, due to the need of American scientists to standardize their medical language and provide a unified method to identify and diagnose mental disorders. Due to the prolific scientific advancement and research being carried out everywhere in the world, the DMS is constantly updated to provide the most reliable and up-to-date information about any given neurological and mental disease. The last version is the DSM-5-TR, developed by the American Psychiatric Society identifies four standards for diagnosing dementia.

Difficulties With Mental Functions

The first parameter to diagnose dementia is verifying whether the patient has an impairment with more than one cognitive task. According to the manual, there are six cognitive domains that could be affected and that need checking. If more than one of the following is impaired, then the first parameter for diagnosing dementia is checked.

If the patient's **complex attention** is disrupted, they will have trouble focusing for long periods, as well as shifting their attention from one target to another. Warning signs of impaired attention are difficulties in maintaining concentration in environments with multiple stimuli (TV, radio, or people speaking simultaneously)

When a person's **executive abilities** are compromised, they will have trouble making plans, problems correcting themselves when making a mistake, or learning from their mistakes. They may stop specific habits belonging to their routine and need help engaging in tasks that require mental flexibility. In practical terms, a patient will need assistance making judgments, will have troubles with organizational tasks (involving their job, for example), and with abstract thinking (having to think of different consequences or outcomes based on a practical problem).

If the patient has issues with their language skills. In that case, they are usually concerned with syntax (arrangement of words and phrases to form proper sentences), grammar, and fluency. In this case, this parameter needs to be carefully monitored because even phrases like "you know what I mean" or using the wrong word with a similar meaning can be indicators of language impairments, which are usually among the first symptoms of dementia.

Another parameter looked at is **memory state**, comprising of short- and long-term memory. Memory is strictly linked with learning because if a person cannot retain information long enough, they will not be able to perform an action based on that. There are many warning signs of this type of impairment, such as not being able to recall recently learned information or shopping lists, engaging in repetitive behavior, and forgetting to do certain things concerning the daily routine.

The patient might also have difficulties with **performing motor or visual tasks**, and signs of this would be difficulties picking things up, orienting in familiar environments, or trouble driving.

The last cognitive ability to be looked at should be **social skills**. This parameter refers to a person's ability to behave appropriately based on the situation, including choosing the right clothes, the topic of conversation, emotional regulation, and inhibition. It also looks at the emotional involvement of a patient in their daily life activities.

So how do doctors and physicians assess all these domains? They certainly don't have the time to observe their patient at home, and simple observation wouldn't be a reliable enough resource. They, instead, use screening tools (tests), and one of the most well-known and widely used is the Montreal Cognitive Assessment Test (MoCA). It's a test with 30 questions, allowing assessment and diagnosis of cognitive impairment along the possible spectrum of disorders. The test contains mental exercises that challenge the cognitive abilities of the patient. For example, there will be images of objects or animals that the person has to name, lists of words to remember and repeat, tasks like drawing a clock with a specific time, and so on.

Decline From Previous Level of Activity

It's important to understand whether the cognitive decline exhibited at the time of diagnosis is new and does not consider skills in which the patient has always been deficient. The MoCa provides an accurate measurement of normal vs. abnormal performance. Out of 30 questions, cognitive decline starts to show up if the patient scores less than 26. However, there might be domains where the patient has always exhibited some degree of difficulty. Tasks like arithmetic, reading a clock, or knowing the meaning of a certain word to remember could be weak spots for specific patients. For this reason, family involvement here is fundamental because it helps the clinician understand whether the exhibited deficits are attributable to a decline or personal characteristics.

Impairment of Activities of Daily Living

After diagnosing possible cognitive decline, the clinician will have to understand if they are severe enough to compromise a person's independence. First of all, what are these daily living activities that a person needs to be able to perform to rule out a possible dementia diagnosis? Simple everyday activities are walking, dressing, feeding, toileting, and moving. The extent to which someone is able to perform these activities independently is an important indicator to start assessing dementia. More complex daily activities are also called instrumental activities and refer to the ability to carry out financial, organizational, housecleaning, and transportation tasks. To get a better idea of what the patient is able to carry out by themselves, the clinician will ask the family to provide an up-to-date report of the patient's level of independence, as well as ask the patient themselves what are the tasks they struggle with and what they feel confident doing.

Presence of possible reversible causes responsible for the cognitive decline

Comorbidity (the presence of two or more diseases affecting the patient) and misdiagnosis are prevalent in the medical world. As we have mentioned earlier, dementia, in particular, has many different but similar conditions that can cause confusion. We've already spoken about the overlap between Mild Cognitive Impairment and dementia. There are other reversible conditions that are even more similar to dementia. One of these conditions is called delirium. Delirium is an acute confusional state usually caused by drug toxicities, dehydration or urinary tract infections (UTI), vitamin deficiencies, sleep deprivation, and a number of other causes. Despite the fact that it can occur at any age, it is most often seen in older people and mainly affects attention rather than other aspects of cognition. After ruling out that the cause of the cognitive impairment is not attributable to delirium or other disorders, including mood disorders, a physician will be closer to diagnosing dementia.

IMPORTANCE AND IMPACT OF EARLY DIAGNOSIS

A diagnosis of dementia usually comes as a bolt from the blue. Many individuals wait for several years before an actual diagnosis is made. During this time, they struggle to understand what is wrong with them, and symptoms usually worsen. Imagine the circumstance where a dementia-affected individual drives a car and engages in other potentially dangerous actions, not knowing how detrimental their behavior is. Consequently, these people are often relieved when they finally obtain their diagnosis, allowing them to make sense of all the struggles they'd gone through before that moment. Having a more thorough look at the benefits of early diagnosis, you'll realize how it can impact your patient and yourself as a caregiver on many different levels. What do we mean by early diagnosis? It refers to the detection of the disease when it is still at stage 2 or 3, which can occur up to eight years before any symptoms show up at all with currently available methods, such as brain scans.

First of all, early diagnosis means early intervention. Due to metabolic and physiological changes, many dementia-affected patients usually experience comorbidities such as diabetes, high cholesterol levels, high blood pressure, obesity, etc. Detecting cognitive decline early enough can also shed light on the potential risk factors of developing those other conditions and develop suitable treatment strategies to intervene. Identifying more than one risk factor for developing dementia is also helpful in identifying early signs. Advanced age, smoking, a sedentary lifestyle, and the APO-E4 gene variant are all risk factors (Rasmussen & Langerman, 2019). If an individual is diagnosed early enough, their life expectancy will significantly increase because they will have access to medication that can slow down the course of the disease.

Second, early diagnosis positively benefits caregivers, too, given their emotional investment during the whole course of the disease. Knowing in advance what to expect, what kind of decline the patient will likely experience, and the extent of care they will have to provide will give them more time to plan ahead in their own life. According to Vugt and Verhey (2013), caregivers who are given enough time to process the diagnosis experience less depression, anxiety, and related psychological difficulties as compared to caregivers who are not given any time before starting their difficult journey.

HOW DIAGNOSIS OCCURS

In the first paragraph of this chapter, we briefly mentioned the main steps to diagnosing dementia, but there is still more to it. First of all, let us clarify the professionals who carry out this diagnosis, so you will know whom to speak with in case of need.

The first person you should address any concern related to the cognitive decline observed in yourself, a family member should be a primary care physician. They are the professionals that deal with any general physical and mental problem who might decide to refer you to another specialist based on the problem they've identified. Some physicians are more familiar with dementia, while others are less, so it's a good idea to ask them about their level of expertise on the matter.

Because dementia diagnosis, as we have seen, is not so easy and straightforward, the help of one or more specialists might be required. Who are these specialists? You should refer to a geriatrician or geriatric psychiatrist, who are primary physicians with extra training and knowledge of age-related conditions. The first are medical doctors who can deal with disorders related to the nervous system and spinal cord. The second one, because they are psychiatrists, can be especially helpful in ruling out other neurological diseases or mental disorders, which is always helpful in determining a dementia diagnosis. Next, neurologists and neuropsychologists are specialists in the nervous system. Neurologists, after obtaining their medical degree, have chosen to specialize in neurology. They might have specific training in certain dementia-related disorders. Neuropsychologists are psychologists who specialize in neurological conditions and are helpful when it comes to administering tests and interpreting them. Last, you have the option of addressing your concerns with a dementia diagnostic center, which usually has multiple specialists to consult and can also determine if the patient meets the criteria to join clinical trials, which may give them the opportunity to access the latest medical treatments.

The mental screening we have described in detail above is sometimes not enough to achieve a proper diagnosis. So, what do specialists do to identify the specific cause of cognitive dysfunction? First, they ask for the patient's medical history to help them identify any risk factors to which the patient might have been exposed. Second, they will perform a physical examination, where blood pressure, temperature, and other parameters are analyzed. In addition, the physicians might also perform other laboratory tests to determine the health of specific organs. These tests include urine and blood samples, cerebrospinal fluid analysis, and so on. Third, screening for depression is always advisable because memory problems and other cognitive slowing can sometimes be attributable to severe depression. Last, and probably most importantly, specific brain scans can further clarify that the symptoms reported are attributable to dementia.

A Computerised Tomography (CT) scan, a type of X-ray that produces images of the brain, may be beneficial because it will detect shrinkage and atrophy, as well as any blood clots or signs of infections. They can also detect signs of damage due to stroke and signs of brain tumors.

Magnetic resonance imaging (MRI), sometimes provides more details than CT scans. MRIs are usually done to discover strokes and blood vessel abnormalities and can help diagnose vascular dementia.

A physician might also choose to perform a Positron Emission Tomography (PET) scan. By injecting non-harmful radioactive dyes which show up in the brain, the dyes bind with the brain molecules and produce very colorful images. PET scans, because they detect molecules rather than provide a clear overall brain image, are particularly helpful in detecting amyloid plaques and tau tangles. PET scans can also show the quality of the brain metabolism, detecting glucose flow.

PART II

CARING ESSENTIALS

"One person caring about another represents life's greatest value."

— JIM ROHN

4

PSYCHOLOGICAL CHANGES

The psychological changes that can occur in a patient with dementia can be very multifaceted. Because their brain is constantly changing, there will be tasks they will not be able to carry out like they used to, and there are a few things you should know to be prepared to face these changes. Remember that such psychological difficulties can be very upsetting and frustrating for them because their perception of relatives and surroundings becomes increasingly confusing daily. This profound confusion arises from the inability of the brain to make sense of the surroundings. The brain's emotional, perceptual, and behavioral spheres no longer communicate as they should.

No dementia-affected patient will exhibit the same symptoms as another, especially when it comes to psychological factors. However, all will show some form of mental health symptom, affecting their behaviors, emotions, and responses. Regardless of dementia, the world of psychiatric and psychological diagnosis faces many challenges due to the overlap between different symptoms and pathologies. In dementia patients, these challenges can be even more problematic because the occurrence of any mental issue can be accompanied by physical difficulties too. Let's examine the main mental challenges that patients can face. To illustrate this, I'll provide scenarios describing the behaviors of a fictional character named Mr. Brown, as seen through the eyes of his caregiver.

DISTURBANCE IN THE EMOTIONAL EXPERIENCE

The first tip I will give you, even before starting to explain psychological changes, is the following:

Brain dysfunctions will cause changes in the patient that you might not understand.

For this reason, you must always keep in mind that behavioral changes are caused by dysfunctional brain mechanisms and not by the patient's will. Remaining calm and always being kind will greatly mitigate these changes. We've already said multiple times that patients experience changes in moods and behavior. But to what extent? These mood shifts are not rare. In fact, it has been estimated that around 50-80% of dementia patients will experience them (Lyketsos et al., 2002). One of the first mood disorders that usually occurs in dementia patients is depression, but it may be expressed in a different way. They may not appear sad or worried but rather completely unmotivated and apathetic. With this type of behavior, they'll exhibit a general loss of interest, and the disturbance will be more towards the spectrum of anxiety, panic, and hypertension. These symptoms might be further expressed with muscle twitches and difficulties in movements.

"When Mr. Brown wakes up, regardless of my efforts to cheer him up and motivate him, he often appears moody and lethargic. During those days, it is tough to engage him in activities, and even harder to carry out activities of daily living (bathing, feeding, etc.)."

These patients will not be apathetic all the time. They will alternate with moments of clarity and cheerfulness, especially during the first stages. Due to the severity of these mood changes, they can impact both the patient and the caregiver. For the latter, it might be particularly challenging to help carry out activities of daily living when the patient is in a state of irritability or an angry outburst. Emotional overreaction is very common in dementia-affected patients. It's usually the result of the patient not understanding and recognizing their surroundings. It represents a defense mechanism to reclaim their lost authority and control over themselves. This lack of understanding might be due to their memory slips, which don't allow them to create a cohesive and coherent structure of events and reality. It can happen with something such as distractedly telling them a task or something you're going to do. "We're going to have a haircut in the afternoon" may not be enough for them to remember the concept. They might only remember a part of that phrase "...in the afternoon" and not understand your action or the hairdresser's action of taking the scissors and bringing them closer to their head.

> *"Early in the morning, I told Mr. Brown that the hairdresser was coming over to give him a haircut, and he agreed. However, that afternoon, when the hairdresser brought the scissors and comb close to his head, he reacted very aggressively and cursed at him."*

In similar cases, the patient might have forgotten who the hairdresser was, and his purpose and might be very ashamed of saying that they forgot (when they understand their memory failed them).

Solutions to handle mood swings and similar situations:

- Always be calm and reassuring: although you are taken aback by certain behaviors, never act shocked and upset. Their unusual reactions to certain events indicate that they are confused and that they do not understand what is going on.
- To deal with difficult days (apathy, low mood), set a daily routine of challenging but pleasurable activities

as early in the caregiving process as possible. This will give them a purpose to get out of bed and may make them be active and happier.

- Never take for granted that they'll remember something you said hours earlier. If you're adding something new and unusual to their routine, remember to talk about it multiple times and listen to their opinion about it.
- Reassure your patient about people and surroundings. Keep in mind that they might be scared and insecure but may not verbalize this.
- If the mood changes become too severe and unmanageable, try to consult support groups or a mental health specialist. Both may be able to provide extra help and solutions.

DELUSIONAL THOUGHTS

Delusional thinking refers to believing something that doesn't hold true. Usually, showing evidence that their conviction is false is not enough to make the patient understand they are wrong. Because delusions involve beliefs, they differ significantly from hallucinations, which are perceptual mistakes and are sensory in nature. A patient might hallucinate an object, a smell, or a voice that is not there. Specific to dementia, common delusions would concern the nature of people. Patients might think that things have been stolen from their house, that people close to them are lying, that others are conspiring against them, or spouses are unfaithful. This thinking pattern is known as paranoia, in which a patient tries to make sense of their confusing surroundings.

> *"Mr. Brown always appears distressed and scared when I lead him to the shower, despite me telling him multiple times that we were going to do that task. I then understood that he was confused because he did not remember ever taking a shower in his own house but that he would always take a bath. The fact that I was forcing him to shower instead (because it was quicker and easier for me) made him believe it wasn't his bathtub or his bathroom and house anymore. He would also think of me as a hostile figure until I began filling the bathtub with water before I brought him into the room."*

Respect your patient's past habits. Abruptly changing them might make them feel scared and insecure. Knowing that this state is very normal in dementia patients should prepare you to face such events with a more aware and positive outlook. Here are a few things that you can do when your patient is being delusional about something.

- Be aware of your tone and choice of words used. Don't take offense: if the patient is being aggressive, it might be because they are troubled by something they believe. Your role, in this case, would be listening to them and calmly reassuring them.

- Eliminate noises and additional people present in the room if possible. Avoid arguing because they will feel attacked and become avoidant. What they believe at that moment is their reality, and telling them they're wrong will just upset and confuse them more.
- Answer their questions in simple terms without making them uncomfortable. If they, for example, ask whether a person has stolen something, you can simply answer, "No, they didn't. They wouldn't do such a thing", and then show them the object.
- After offering reassurance, try to switch the focus of attention, engaging them in a different and entertaining activity, such as going to another room or for a walk.

PERCEPTUAL DISTURBANCES OR HALLUCINATIONS

You should be aware that some types of dementia cause perceptual hallucinations in people affected by it. When the parts of the brain involved in visual perception and identification get damaged during the course of the disease, your patient might not see the world in the same way in which they used to. For example, if a patient has damage to their parietal or temporal lobes. They might have issues recognizing faces or objects. In some cases, the hallucinations are more severe and might lead individuals to see things that were never really there. This happens mainly with Lewy body and Parkinson's dementia, but it can happen with Alzheimer's too. Lewy body dementia is the most severe in this matter. This type of dementia can cause patients to see vivid things like animals or human figures. They can also have olfactory hallucinations. One in ten people with this dementia will smell scents and odors that aren't really there (Team, 2021). As you might imagine, this experience can be very frightening and debilitating, making the person unsure and often scared about their surroundings. If this repeatedly happens to your patient, you might want to address the issue with their doctor, as they might prescribe different medications. To understand whether a patient is having hallucinations, you should pay attention to any unusual behaviors.

"I would sometimes spot Mr. Brown suspiciously looking out of the window. Other times, I would see him wandering around the house as if he was looking for something or someone."

Very common hallucinations involve seeing weird things out of the window or people in the house (either strangers or people belonging to their past). When this happens, your patient might choose not to tell you because they might realize how strange what they saw was. Ignoring such unusual behaviors is not a good solution.

However, don't forget about the possible presence of other conditions in dementia-affected patients, such as eye-sight and hearing loss. What might resemble the worrying sign of a hallucination might simply be the result of vision problems or a decrease in hearing. In this case, a patient might think that people entered the house simply by hearing muffled voices coming from the tv. They might mistakenly see something in the mirror or the corners of the room due to shadows or vision issues. Before deciding that your patient is hallucinating, make sure that what they are seeing or hearing is not the result of a sensory *mistake*, which can be verified by an eye-sight or hearing test.

Whenever you notice that your patient is having a vivid hallucination, you can try the following tips.

1. Decide if you need to respond to the hallucination. If it's not upsetting or causing them distress, don't respond or call attention to the fact that it's not there. Don't pretend you can see what they see, though. Let them know you don't see what they see, but you believe them. They may see a bluebird on the windowsill. You can say, "you've always enjoyed looking out the window and watching the birds."

2. Listen to the patient as they describe their hallucination for two reasons.

  1. Making them feel listened to will immediately make them feel calmer.
  2. It will give you the opportunity to formulate a reasonable and logical answer to prove their hallucination isn't real. "You can't be seeing a cat

because the door has been closed all day," rather than simply telling them they are wrong.

3. While you explain, try to show the patient that what they're seeing is not there by leading them to the exact point of the hallucination if it is not too upsetting.

4. If what they are seeing is unreachable and abstract, gently remove the patient from the room where they are hallucinating and lead them somewhere else.

5. Try to move the focus of their attention and engage them in another activity until they become calm and confident.

6. Learn their triggers. Perhaps you will observe that your patient experiences more hallucinations when the tv is on or when a particular window is open. Maybe the sun is shining in and creating a reflection, or a mirror is reflecting an object or person in another room. Take the time to observe their environment and try to prevent their hallucinations by removing their triggers.

By contrast, avoid doing these things.

- Avoid arguing with your patient. Using verbal explanations will not work. When they experience a hallucination, they're frightened and deeply convinced about the integrity of what they are seeing. Arguing with them will also decrease the trust they have in you.

- Avoid playing along. It's no use pretending that you see or hear what they do. Hallucinations only last for a little while. When they return to reality and stop seeing or hearing what they were before, realizing you were reinforcing their initial belief will only worsen the situation.
- Don't ever underestimate and minimize their struggle. Remember, you are their anchor, and they'll need your psychological comprehension and support.

PERSONALITY CHANGES

Emotional changes and the occurrence of hallucinations and delusions will, in one way or another, cause changes in personality too. In normal conditions, many parts of our brain contribute to creating our personality. With dementia and neuronal loss, those brain areas are compromised, deeply modifying behavior and the person's temperament. The frontal lobes, for example (see Figure 2), are very much responsible for directing our attention, planning ahead, and rationally integrating our emotions. For example, linking a meaning to a feeling (feeling of happiness paired with eating ice cream). When dementia kills the neurons of this brain area, a person might become more passive, more restless, and generally less motivated and organized. Based on this, the following tip should always be present in your mind.

Brain changes will cause personality changes, regardless of your patient's will.

Aggressiveness and irritability might be side effects of these brain changes. The patient might feel frustrated and confused about not being able to do simple things. The presence of hallucinations and delusions might further exacerbate their feelings, making them feel more insecure about their relatives and surroundings. Don't forget that, along with psychological changes, patients also undergo profound and often painful physical changes too. Because of this, they might also feel irritable for not being able to communicate their physical discomforts and difficulties, which, in turn, might cause extra pain. Due to their inability to make sense of their feelings during confusional states, they might rely on you to understand how to behave. *Just like a child mirrors their parents' behavior, your patient might reflect your personality and way of being.* This means that if you are irritable and worried, they might behave in the same way, simply because they need a reference point to know how to behave.

As a good caregiver and observer, there are a few things you can do to help your patient and yourself as you take this journey together.

- Try to keep track of their behavior (keeping a written log is helpful). Check to see if it follows a pattern or if it changes abruptly. Based on what you observe, report it to their health care provider because it might be a symptom of a medication's side effects or pain that the patient might struggle to communicate.

- Some medications are used to improve behavioral changes, but they're not always the answer to everything. Because of increasing doses and the adverse side effects that some can have, relying only on medication might not work.

- Just like a child crying to communicate a need, your patient might protest and act aggressively to make you aware of something that is troubling them. Learn to understand their code language, which can take many different forms.

- Observing their behaviors also means identifying any trigger or root cause. A specific person or activity might trouble your patient based on many different factors. If, for example, you realize that a particular person makes your patient irritable and upset, try to prepare your patient to meet that person. This might help the patient get used to them and change their attitude with time.

- Understand the nature and consequences of their behavior. Your role as a caregiver is also to make sure that your patient is safe and doesn't engage in risky behavior. If the personality changes don't cause any harm to themselves or others (walking around the house, talking alone, playing games), then you don't need to change anything as long as they make your patient comfortable. If, on the other hand, you notice harmful behaviors (leaving the house alone, harming themselves with objects, harming others), you'll need to intervene by distracting them.

- Dealing with personality changes can be mentally challenging and physically tiring. As a consequence, knowing when to take a break is fundamental to taking care of your health too. Identify some key activities that calm you down, and always try to take some time for yourself.

- If you're unable to leave home due to the nature of your role as a caregiver, don't underestimate the value of online support groups. Support groups are always there to help. Speaking with other caregivers might give you new perspectives and solutions that you might not have considered before.

Now, let's talk about a more practical approach to some specific difficulties you might encounter.

5

PHYSICAL CHANGES

If dealing with the psychological difficulties of your patient seems hard, physical changes can be even more challenging both for you and for them. Sometimes it might get so unmanageable that you wish your innermost secret desire would come true: to stop being a caregiver. Knowing what's going on in your patient's mind and how to deal with their emotional struggles is not enough. Dealing with a dementia patient means much more than that, and it includes knowing what to expect from their bodies too. Let's take a closer look.

BRAIN AND BODY CONNECTION

When we spoke about the brain, we mainly mentioned how it allows us to perform cognitive abilities like speaking, reasoning, remembering, and thinking. When you think about the brain, those abilities might be some of the first ones which come to mind. However, you must not forget that the brain is involved in many other body functions and is responsible for the physiology of your organism. The way your body works and is kept in balance is highly determined by the functioning of your brain. In normal conditions, we see a cognitive and physical decline in older adults because as the brain ages, it cannot perform certain tasks flawlessly. In dementia patients, this condition is further worsened by quicker neuronal cell death and slowing of the brain altogether. Let's focus on what you, as a caregiver, should expect in practical terms so that you feel more confident and capable in your job. Always remember that your help is fundamental. Knowing that a physical difficulty can occur before it becomes visible may prevent your patient from getting hurt and help you consider resources that may help.

Loss of Coordination and Balance

Because the brain slowly loses more and more cells, it will eventually start losing those controlling motor abilities. Your patient will begin having issues with coordination when the brain stops communicating with its limbs as it used to. This will make finger, hand, and leg coordination particularly harder, requiring your help in specific activities of daily living. Importantly, when this starts to occur, it can initially go unnoticed.

"As the days passed, I noticed that Mr. Brown was losing interest in some of the things he used to love the most. He suddenly stopped cooking, watching TV, and working with puzzles. When I asked him to help me set the kitchen table, he suddenly sounded irritated and upset. After questioning him about his feelings and physical symptoms, I understood that he couldn't use his hands to do those things anymore."

Here are some physical changes you can expect and some tips to help with these challenges:

Balance Issues

Loss of balance can be dangerous to the patient and you as the caregiver. Should you try to catch the patient, or if the patient falls on you or interferes with your balance, they could cause you to fall. Taking walks and exercising may help your loved one remain active and maintain their balance. Not to mention, a walk outside is good for you as well. Some exercises to do with your loved one are heel and toe exercises that you can do together. With heel exercises, you and your loved one will each stand behind a sturdy chair (side by side so the patient can copy you) and lift your heels. Do this exercise 10 times. You will do the same thing for the toe exercises but lift the toes ten times. These can be done seated as well. You can also have your loved one stand behind the chair, holding on to each side and stand on one leg. To do this, lift the left leg by bending it at the knee and hold for 5 to 10 seconds. Repeat with the right leg. You can also try putting a piece of tape or using an imaginary line and have your loved one walk heel to toe on the line. You should lightly place your hands on each side or on their shoulders to help steady them some. If they are too wobbly, don't do this exercise. To help reduce falls, you should make sure all paths are clear of cords, throw rugs, and any other items that can be tripped over. Many insurances cover all or most of the costs for Home Health Care in the home. These companies can provide in-home physical therapy to help with balance. They also have registered nurses, speech therapists, occupational therapists, and medical social workers too.

Shuffling or dragging feet

There are a number of reasons dementia patients begin dragging or shuffling their feet. There could have been a fall or near fall, making them fearful, difficulties with seeing, pain in hips or legs, arthritis, or poorly fitting shoes. Again, some stretching, exercises, and movement may help with muscle weakness and with this behavior. Chair Yoga and other exercises are good to incorporate here as well. Something as simple as a new pair of shoes and talking with the patient may alleviate the issue. Also, discuss with your physician in case it's a side effect of a medication.

Trouble standing or sitting

In the long run, difficulty with standing or sitting might make them inactive and sedentary. To avoid this, try providing them with a tall, steadier armrest-equipped chair. It will support the arms and raise their balance point, which means they will need to bend their knees less to stand up and sit down. There are also lift chairs, but that is not always an option when many caregivers have stopped working to care for their loved one. Grab bars in key locations such as the bathroom and possibly by the bed, and raised toilet seat can help too.

How caregivers can help

- Encourage exercise
- Provide healthy foods
- Care for their skin
- Do passive range of motion exercises with them
- Have a physical therapist come to the home to help

Weak or stiff muscles

While muscle weakness and stiffness can occur in anyone as they age, this condition is further worsened by dementia, making it even more painful and harder to handle. The brain's cell death can also cause rigidity, making it hard to initiate movements. Muscle stiffness can cause cramping and pain because it feels as if the muscle itself is tight and cannot be contracted or elongated. If you are unsure whether your patient is in pain and they cannot properly communicate with you, you could use a face chart. This method consists of showing your patient different facial expressions paired with an emotion related to the feeling of pain. (The chart may not work for patients in the later stages of the disease.)

When you finally figure out the location of the pain, here are a few things you can do to help your loved one.

- Try to motivate your patient to move and exercise. This will keep the body and muscles active and make stiffness less likely to occur. Forcing them to move will be of no help here: why would they do something that causes them pain and discomfort? This is a time when, again, physical therapy or occupational therapy can help. I've often seen a patient participate with a therapist when they wouldn't work with the caregiver.
- Massage can help when they don't feel like moving. You can try putting some pressure with your fingers on the areas that hurt. This can ease the pain when your patient is tired and unmotivated.

Fatigue and problems sleeping

Many dementia patients experience fatigue as the disease progresses. As the brain continues to deteriorate, they may find it more tiring, even exhausting, to do the most simple tasks. Eating or even keeping up with what is going on in their surroundings can be difficult. Another very detrimental physical change occurring in dementia patients is the reduction of sleep quality, which is a fundamental task that normal brains carry out. A brain area called the suprachiasmatic nucleus (which is located inside the hypothalamus) regulates the sleep-wake cycle also known as the circadian rhythm.

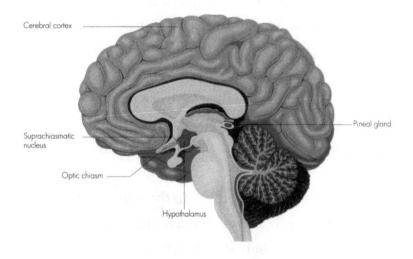

Due to the progressive cell death in dementia patients, this brain area is unable to distinguish day from night, causing the individual to sleep sporadically during the day and gradually less during the night. Because the patient might avoid telling you about their sleep problems, it's important that you keep an eye on them during the day to detect any signs of stress due to sleep deprivation.

Dementia-affected people might start wanting to do things during the night. They don't realize what time of the day it is, and they feel restless. They might want to cook, wander around the house, or even go out. If you notice some of these behaviors or suspect that your patient is having trouble sleeping, here are a few tips for you.

- Keep them active during the day so that they get tired by bedtime. Anything that can healthily keep the body active during the day will be of much help to keep them awake. Engaging them in activities, taking them for a car ride, or going for a walk helps.
- Limit caffeine, limit fluid intake an hour before bedtime, and make sure they have used the bathroom before going to sleep. If appropriate, introduce a night light or make sure the room is dark and comfortable enough.
- If they wake up at night, speak to them in a calm and quiet voice. Gently remind them it's night and wait for them to sleep again. If this happens frequently, add a latch to the top of the entry/exit doors, so they don't wander out when you're asleep. When installing a latch, don't bring it to your loved one's attention, lest they may be more likely to try to unlatch it when you're not watching.

Difficulty with bladder and bowels

Another extremely debilitating issue with dementia, often beginning in the middle stages of the disease, is urinary and bowel incontinence. This frailty is usually associated with difficulty remembering where the bathroom is, how to behave in a bathroom, and, during later stages, no longer feeling the physical urgency. Dementia patients in their last stages will progressively need more and more help until they are entirely dependent on their caregiver in order to perform such tasks. Incontinence can be caused by a variety of reasons, such as bladder infection or weakening, sphincter dysfunction, and so on. Keep in mind that some cases of urinary incontinence can be treated with medication. so speak with a doctor to see if this would be a solution for your loved one. If the physician cannot recommend any medications, here are some tips.

- Consider using a protective pad, especially if the incontinence only causes some leaking. This might help your patient feel more confident in public settings and with themselves. You can try absorbent underwear if your patient struggles to wear protective pads.
- Dress in comfortable and protective clothing. Rather than dressing your patient in uncomfortable zippered trousers, opt for pull-on trousers or skirts with elastic waistbands or anything that feels more soothing for your patient.
- Make the bathroom safer and more visible. Because patients might forget where the bathroom is, try to keep the door open and the lights on. Put some stickers on the door so that it catches your patient's attention. As for safety, make sure that the room has all the necessary tools and items to make your

patient feel safe: grab bars, raised toilet seat, a clear floor, accessible light, and so on.

- If the above-mentioned are not enough, and your patient needs extra assistance, try to help them with verbal instructions while they carry out their tasks. Simply describing the correct steps to them may help them accomplish the task.

- Your patient might feel embarrassed to ask for help. Watch for any signs of needing to go to the bathroom, such as irritability or restlessness. Ask them if they need to go every time before they go to bed.

- Remember, toileting accidents are going to happen. Stay calm and understand that your loved one is not choosing to make more work for you. Being prepared, protecting furniture, and having a plan before your patient gets to this stage will help with some of the stress of this stage of the disease.

You should always strive to preserve your patient's dignity and well-being. Never try to make them feel ashamed, and always remember that their issues are beyond their will and their control.

Skin breakdown

As the disease progresses and the patient begins having trouble toileting, skin breakdown can be an issue. Left untreated, it can be highly detrimental to the patient's overall health. You'll find that, at this point, you'll be caring for your loved one as if they were your child. Here are some things to do to prevent skin breakdown.

Keep skin clean and dry.

- Try to have a bathroom schedule so that there are fewer accidents and that skin exposure to urine and stool matter will be less frequent.
- Use a moisture barrier after cleaning. The moisture barrier protects from sweat, urine, and stool matter.
- Change clothing/briefs as soon as possible, so that urine and stool are quickly removed from the skin.
- If a patient cannot move and change positions, they should be placed in a different position or turned every couple of hours to alleviate pressure on certain areas that can cause bedsores. Use special care in areas such as the tailbone, hips, heels, or elbows. These areas are sensitive and at high risk for tears and breakdown. Use disposable briefs. Also, please keep in mind that the term "adult diaper" and "diaper" are less dignified than "briefs".

Sundowning

As dementia patients struggle with their sleep pattern disturbances, they are also affected by another phenomenon: sundowning. This refers to a drastic mood change that occurs when the sun goes down and continues throughout the evening and sometimes night too. The most common sundowning symptoms are agitation, irritability, anxiety, restlessness, delusions, hallucinations, discomfort, and detachments. Sundowning can have a variety of causes, such as accumulated stress during the day, but the exact roots are not well known. You may also notice that your patient may have sundowning behavior one day but not the next. Here are a few things that can help in managing these symptoms.

- While scheduling a regular daily routine to keep wake and bedtimes in balance, it's also essential that your patient is exposed to as much natural night as possible. To do this, take them regularly on outside walks, possibly in parks or quiet places.
- Avoid coffee, tea, or any other stimulant two to four hours before bedtime, which can help facilitate sleep.
- To get them back into a regular sleep pattern, expose them to Light Therapy during the morning. This involves sitting one to two feet away from a source of artificial light to trick the body into thinking it's natural light. The light will signal the body to stop producing the sleep hormone called melatonin and will regulate the circadian rhythm. You should consult a doctor and use a light therapy box designed to serve that purpose.
- If your patient starts having sundowning behavior all of a sudden, you should consult the doctor. Other factors could contribute to the behavior, such as

infection, dehydration, or a medication dosage change.

Other Behavioral Changes

Shadowing - following a partner or caregiver around

Because dementia patients usually feel insecure and lost, it's very common that they choose to follow their caregiver because they're the only reference in a world of confusion. In the middle to later stages of dementia, you may start noticing some clingy and other unusual behaviors, like pacing, repeating things, asking the same questions over and over, and following you around. These things can be annoying, but showing them you're annoyed will only make things worse. Try to keep calm and identify the correct strategy for both of you to be happy. Take notice of what's going on in their surroundings. Are they doing these things at a certain time of day? Are there things in the home different, less organized, or new? Is it noisy, or do you have visitors over? Have you asked the patient to do something that they don't want to do? Here are some solutions for dealing with these behaviors.

- If they're following you while you're doing chores, ask them to help you and give them a task. Reassure them and let them know they're safe. Talk about a period in their life in which they were happy. It's not necessary to tell them a spouse or loved one has moved on. If they bring this up, change the conversation to events during the time they were with that person and talk about other positive things that happened at that time in their life. Listening to music and eliminating any excess noise is helpful too.

Repetitive Behavior

Saying the same thing, doing the same thing, and asking the same question over and over can be very hard (sometimes maddening) to deal with as a caregiver. Remember, you need patience here.

Evaluate what the trigger may be for this behavior. Does your loved one think that they're lost? Assure them that they're safe. If they ask the same question repeatedly, it's very likely they don't remember saying or doing what they've just done. Remember, they are not trying to annoy you. They simply can't remember. Ask them some questions about something they like to talk about or used to like to do. For repeated questions of "when are we going to a particular place/appointment," repeatedly asking what time it is or that they need to be at a particular place, gently reassure them that you will make sure they get to the right place on time.

Help them find the answer for themselves. I've known caregivers who purchased an AI device such as Alexa, Cortana, Echo, or Siri just for this reason. A calendar, a talking clock, or a timepiece that displays the day, date, and time are also helpful if these are some of the questions that are repeated. A fidget blanket or fidget box may be beneficial for patients who wring their hands or zip and unzip zippers. The blankets have zippers, pockets, buttons, etc., that may help with repetitive behavior. Small puzzles with big pieces are excellent fidget items, as are a deck of cards.

Use a shoebox (or several different ones) and fill it with fidget items. Here are some ideas of what to use.

- Wooden Beads
- Fuzzy balls
- Spikey balls *
- Squishy stress balls
- Short pieces of yarn
- Long pieces of string that you've started a ball with
- Old Keys on a keyring
- Velcro pieces that are stuck together
- Stickers/sticker books
- wooden puzzles, shape match, block puzzles (like for kids)
- Word search puzzles (if appropriate)
- Pieces of an old button-up shirt with buttons intact to button and unbutton
- Pieces of memory foam
- Playdough
- Small stuffed animals/dolls

Memory Boxes are also helpful for some Dementia patients. Make sure, for a memory box, that you focus on items that will remind your patient of joyous times. Some examples are:

- Photos of loved ones - labeled
- Souvenirs from vacation trips - marked with the place
- Old ticket stubs from events attended
- Jewelry
- Old Letters
- Old work items or ID cards from work.
- Collector cards, like baseball cards
- Seashells
- Scented items like soap
- Old Coins
- Postcards
- Old newspaper clippings

Loss of Interest in Activities and with Friends

In the earlier stages of dementia, you may notice your loved one avoiding activities and not going places they previously went. This may be because they feel less confident in their cognitive abilities. Understand that this can be a very difficult time for them. Encourage them to continue things they've enjoyed in the past. There may be a few changes they need to make, like going to events with smaller groups of people. Tell them where they're going, and let them know who they'll be seeing. The patient will likely have trouble coping with large, loud events, but keeping things simple will help them with this transition.

Stealing Things

Most of the time, dementia-affected people are unaware of their surroundings, the reason for which they might engage in inappropriate behavior. Stealing things from stores is very common because they may forget to pay or even that they're in a store. There are a few things you can do to avoid this from occurring.

- Avoid having them wear clothes with pockets.
- If they do have pockets, check them before leaving the store.
- Keep an eye on them all the time, and if you see them stealing something, remember to gently explain to them what they have done wrong rather than scold them.
- Ask your doctor to write a disclaimer that your patient has dementia to justify their behavior. Also, have business-size cards that you can hand to someone (on the card, it will say this person has Dementia)

In this chapter, you've learned some useful tips to manage the problematic physical complications that can arise from a debilitating illness like dementia. Whenever you are feeling exhausted or annoyed by a certain behavior or task, just remember how frustrating it must feel for them. Preserving their dignity is the most important thing, and you should never make them feel ashamed. However, being a caregiver is harder than it sounds, and looking after your mental and physical health matters too. We'll talk about that very soon.

6

COPING WITH DIFFICULT SITUATIONS

"What you do speaks so loud that I cannot hear what you say."

— RALPH WALDO EMERSON

Dementia is complex and multifaceted. You will often be confronted with even more difficult situations, some of which may make you feel as if you are at the end of your rope. This book is here to remind you that there is a solution for everything. You just need to know where to look.

7 WAYS TO COMBAT BEHAVIOR ISSUES

Let's start with the assumption that there's always a reason for someone's behavior, and dementia patients are no exception. During your journey toward understanding your patient's behavior, you should always maintain a positive outlook and a gentle approach. Arguing won't lead anywhere. As the cognitive abilities of your patient start declining, they will be progressively less able to understand their own behavior. For example, imagine that you're having a rough day and suddenly snap at a member of your family. Because your cognitive abilities are intact, you would be able to understand the root cause of your behavior and perhaps apologize to the person. Your dementia patient, on the other hand, doesn't necessarily understand the reasons for which they do or say certain things, and part of your job is to make sense of their mood changes. The following actions are aimed at trying to understand specific unexplainable reactions your patient may demonstrate. Let's go over what steps to follow and how they can be beneficial for you.

1. Reassuring

Before even trying to understand your patient's behavior, you should focus on establishing a relationship of mutual trust and respect. Since dealing with them will be difficult most of the time, you should start considering dementia as a third existing entity causing all the troubles and stop blaming your patients for what they do.

"Mr. Brown was convinced that his deceased wife was still alive and cheating on him with the neighbor. He would shout and curse at him whenever he saw him from his window. He got so obsessed with it that he started staring out of his window all day, every day."

Instead of reacting aggressively to similar behavior, try to empathize with the patient and think how hurtful it must feel to believe that your wife is still alive and cheating on you. So, what can you do to reassure your patient?

- Before trying to reassure someone, you should make sure your frustration is in check and you are calm enough. If you approach them when you are annoyed and upset, it will only panic them more and make them feel insecure and unlistened to. Take a moment for yourself before going to talk to them, and think about the fact that it's their dementia making them behave in a certain way.
- When someone falls prey to a delusion, a hallucination, or even a simple suspicion - as can happen to anyone during daily life, (e.g., feeling that a partner is cheating is not exclusive to dementia patients), they need to know that a friend is there to help and support them. Telling them, they are loved, that no one would ever do any harm to them and that they are protected is key to damper any feeling of anger they might feel. Always approach a

dementia patient who's upset from the front, walk slowly and talk calmly to them. Make sure your body language conveys what you're saying.

- Acknowledge the emotional value of their experience. Whether they are upset, withdrawn, or clingy (following you around all the time), just know that they are living in a moment of great emotional confusion and don't know how to react other than what they're doing. Don't say "calm down," as this will not help the situation. You should respond to the emotion they are experiencing, not the behavior they are displaying.

2. Understand Underlying Causes

Start acknowledging that their behaviors are not done purposefully to upset you. A person needs to engage in highly cognitive mechanisms to plan an upsetting behavior on purpose, and dementia patients don't have the mental capacities. Instead, their behaviors reflect coping mechanisms for things around them they can't explain.

"Whenever Mr. Brown would sit and wait for his deceased wife and not see her return, he would then start obsessing with the fact that she was cheating on him. He would wake up and be mad at her: he would wait for her for hours and hours, and it was heartbreaking to watch."

Most of their behaviors reflect ways that their confused brain has sorted to explain external phenomena that they struggle to understand. Explaining the disappearance of things with theft, misunderstandings, miscommunications met with hostility, and so on. Now, reading the theory doesn't always teach what to do in practical terms, so here are the tips to try.

- Gently ask your patient questions to understand their feelings, thoughts, and behavior. For example, if they are hurting and are lashing out due to pain, you'll be able to recognize this as a factor in the behavior if it happens again.
- Think about the timing and what may be different. Are they tired from a poor night's sleep? Is there more noise than usual? Are there visitors over they don't remember or know? Maybe they're hungry or have to use the bathroom. Are they frustrated with trying to do something?
- Finding a pattern to their behavior will help you prevent future reoccurrences from happening. For example, if you notice that a certain reaction is initiated at a particular time of the day, you'll be more careful the next day at the same time and try to engage your patient in different activities.

3. Identify and Remove Triggers

Sometimes, some behaviors are caused by specific objects or people that can trigger your patient. In the case of Mr. Brown, the question you should ask yourself to identify the trigger is, what causes him to believe that his wife is still alive in the first place? Is he looking in his closet and seeing his wife's clothes? Is there anything in the house that reminds him of his wife? In this case, as in every similar circumstance, the goal should be removing the patient from the trigger before they are exposed to it. Generally speaking, remember to

- Remove all the objects from the patient's sight that remind them of an upsetting or discomforting event.
- Free their room from any object that can trigger delusions or hallucinations. A weird-shaped object could project a frightening shadow and scare your patient, preventing them from sleeping.
- Also remove "activity triggers." For example, a particular sound or event might remind them to do something they were doing earlier in their life. The sound of an alarm might warn them they must go to work (as they used to), initiating potentially dangerous behaviors such as leaving the house unattended. In a similar situation, removing the alarm and distracting them during that time of the day would divert their attention. We are exploring this further in step number

4. Redirect Attention

The best way to redirect someone's attention is to engage them in activities that make them feel helpful. Rather than simply telling them to focus on something else, start doing something and show them you are having a hard time (anything from cooking, crafting, folding clothes, or tidying up the house). Be dramatic! Show them you're dropping things and messing around, and then tell them, "Mr. Brown, I really need your help!" Making them feel needed will substantially increase your chances of catching their attention and shifting the object of focus. Here are some other ideas to redirect your loved one.

- Offer different choices among the things they enjoy the most. "Would you rather go to the park or bake brownies with me?" They'll be thrilled by the choice while being very excited about both things. If they're at a stage where choices upset them, ask a yes or no question. Do you want to go for a walk in the park?
- Start a conversation about cheerful events belonging to their past. This will literally take them back in time and potentially have them relieve those events. Be careful, however, not to mention anything triggering for them (the death of a relative, for example). Don't ask, "do you remember," use a phrase like, "you used to like working in the garden," or "you can grow the prettiest tomatoes."

- Move them to a different location with phrases like "I want to show you something," will you come with me? Make it sound exciting and intriguing.
- Get their memory box and start telling them about the things in the box.

5. Take care of yourself

Don't ever forget that you're the solid rock of the duo and, for this reason, you must look after yourself more than ever. If you surrender, your patient will also surrender, so it's important that you take some time to refuel and renew your strength, patience, and inner peace. What are the things you can do to take care of yourself?

- Meditation is the act of focusing entirely on your inner self, feelings, and emotions by letting out all the negativity. Engaging in 15-minutes of daily meditation can help vent and release all the negative energies. This can be done in yoga classes, but there are plenty of online courses made specifically for people who cannot leave their homes for long periods of time. It may be something you haven't tried before, but it's worth a shot.
- Take the time to do the things you really enjoy. Once or twice a week, arrange a visit from another family member or friend to your patient, and during that time, go for a walk, see your friends or do anything that makes you happy. Choose a time of the day

when you know that your patient is more manageable and give instructions to the visitor. Even an hour or two can really make a difference;

- If you cannot leave your patient unattended, there are a variety of services that can be offered at home, such as hairdressers, personal trainers, grocery store deliveries, and much more. You deserve your dose of self-care, too, and never underestimate its importance.

- You must hydrate and take care to eat properly. Drink plenty of water and make sure you have nutritious meals. Many times, a caregiver will skip meals because they're exhausted and just not hungry but you must give your body the nutrition it needs.

- Keep a diary or journal. Writing down your feelings can help, and you can express emotions that you may not be able to voice.

- Take deep, relaxing breaths.

- Have a visitor come sit for an hour and a half with your loved one. While they're visiting, light a candle or turn on a scented diffuser in your room, put a face mask or lotion on your face, soak in the tub for 30 minutes, stretch out and listen to music, an audiobook or watch your favorite show for 30 minutes uninterrupted.

- Treat yourself! Bake your favorite dessert or meal or order food delivery or takeout.

- Forgive yourself! You've been thrust into a position you probably weren't prepared for at a time when you didn't expect this to happen. You'll have a roller coaster of emotions. It's ok to be angry, sad and hurt, and it's ok to say you don't want to do this! It's something many of us must endure whether we want to or not.

6. Mentally Record What Happened

Life is a constant learning experience, so why would we live anything in the first place if we didn't have the ability to learn from it? Any anger outburst or unusual and annoying behavior is an opportunity to get to know your patient better. In fact, you cannot get to know someone by simply reading a manual; new mothers might learn the basics of childbearing and care by reading a book but will not learn how to understand their child as a person. Each individual has their own history, personality, and identity, and you should focus on learning their new traits if you want to learn how to manage their behavior. To do that, mentally record what happened during the day, what upset them, and what made them happy, so you will be able to understand how to please them and avoid upsetting them in the future.

"After I started observing Mr. Brown's preferences and passions, I soon understood that he liked chocolate brownies and western movies. What seemed to be unimportant details soon revealed to be game changers in my caring journey: I

would wake him up with his favorite brownies and propose
to watch a western movie every other night. He was happier
and more relaxed."

Targeting their passions might be a game-changer, but
mentally recording their negative reactions might be helpful
too. Understanding what triggered a specific response,
studying their behavior, and so on will make you learn how
to avoid its reoccurrence, how to react, and what to expect in
the future. In particular, there are two things that can help
you prevent disruptive behaviors.

- Set a routine. This will give a mental structure to
  your patient, who will have less opportunities to
  behave in unexpected ways. If they're used to having
  their meal at 1 pm and know it's time for their daily
  walk at 1:30, then try to adhere to that schedule.
- Exercise. Keeping your patient physically and
  mentally active can make their mood happier. For
  example, if you know you need a couple of hours to
  do house chores, engage them in a different activity
  every time you change rooms. Instead of placing
  them in front of a tv all day, having them help can
  burn off extra energy and make them more tired,
  which can aid in sleep.

7. Ask for Help When Needed

As a dementia caregiver, you will soon learn at your expense that behaviors and reactions can't always be predicted. Many different variables are at play when it comes to dealing with difficult behaviors. Sometimes your patient will do things that they've never done before, and you'll find yourself in a situation where fast thinking and reacting are required. You must accept that you can't always deal with everything by yourself. There might be times when your patient doesn't recognize you and will try to hit you or might react aggressively to something you've done. In such cases, no matter how stable and prepared you are, you need a hand to manage the situation. Reach out to online and local dementia support groups. Don't be afraid to ask for help and look after your own mental health. If you notice that your sleep quality has declined due to your patient's sleep issues, make sure that a doctor addresses this issue with your patient. You may not want to medicate, but it's sometimes necessary when you're experiencing aggressive behavior from your patient.

Other behavioral Issues

Aggressive, Impulsive & Threatening behavior

Unexpected behavior can also become very hard and sometimes dangerous to handle. If your patient is behaving aggressively all of a sudden, you'll want to try and understand the root cause in order to find a solution.

*"There were days when Mr. Brown would start answering
my questions very frantically and aggressively. Once,
because I asked him to repeat something twice, he smashed
his glass on the door, missing my face for only a few inches.
I got really scared."*

Unpleasant episodes can happen, and before they become a frequent occurrence, you should apply the following tips to try and determine what is causing them.

- Your patient might be in physical pain, and the anger might rise from their difficulty or inability to communicate with you. If you think this is the case, or even to rule out this possibility, call a doctor, and have them do a general check to identify a possible cause for their pain.
- The patient might react in a certain way because they haven't properly slept for a few days, something you might not have noticed if you were sleeping. Start monitoring their sleeping pattern by placing a baby monitor beside their bed. This might wake you if they're up and allow you to help them fall asleep again.
- You could also ask your doctor to review the medications the patient is taking and assess the possibility of any side effects. Progressively lowering the dose of a medicine, strictly under the supervision

of their doctor, might decrease the severity of side effects, if any exist.

In the meantime, make sure you take care that their surroundings are not unpleasant, noisy, untidy, or upsetting. Through observation, you might understand that the amount of light in the house is troubling them or specific objects are triggering their anger.

Anxiety Related To Dementia

Anxious behaviors can come from a variety of different reasons, and the root causes are usually incomprehensible. However, try to think for a moment about the level of cognitive burden your patient is subject to every day. Life becomes very demanding for them, and they are constantly confronted with the pressure of doing the simplest things, which are now hard and unmanageable. Progressively, even going to the toilet or completing a task becomes complicated, and their psychological health suffers from it. One simple thing you can try to help with their anxiety is to decrease the number of things they have to do. If a specific task, something you have told them to do to keep them active, is particularly demanding and challenging, make sure they get enough mental rest before engaging them in something else. Their daily routine shouldn't be a boot camp to train their cognitive skills; it should be engaging just enough, so they don't feel bored and lonely. Avoid forcing them into doing things they don't want to do. Here are some practical and useful tips for you to help your patient fight off anxiety.

- Use positive language even when the task they have completed could be done better. For example, if your patient had to fold some clothes but has done it in a sloppy manner, try saying, "Well done! Rather than saying, "No, you've done it wrong."
- Use a reward system. Make sure that they see the benefits of being active. You might say, "If you walk with me to the shop, I can make that stew you love so much!" or "If you help me clean the house up, I can invite your friend over! Give them a reason for doing something, and you may see a change in their attitude.

Apathy

This mental condition is something with which the majority of dementia patients struggle. It's exhibited as a lack of motivation and initiation, poor engagement, and generally a lack of interest in things and people. It is usually the result of a phenomenon called "learned helplessness," for which individuals see that they fail multiple times in their tasks and progressively lose hope for their success. They slowly give up as a mechanism to cope with the frustration of not succeeding. The more apathetic a patient is, the more the burden will be on the caregiver to perform activities of daily living, which might lead to extreme stress and strain for the caregiver. There are a few things you can do to minimize these sorts of occurrences.

- Don't overwhelm your patient. Introduce one change at a time. Changing routine might be beneficial and stimulating, but if you do it too quickly or abruptly, you might risk overloading your patient, causing the opposite reaction.
- Develop a challenging environment where the patient is inspired and motivated. Again, gently introduce the things they like, giving them the possibility to choose between different tasks when possible.
- Always be gentle and never scold your patient when they don't manage to do something. This might exacerbate their feelings of worthlessness and worsen their apathy.
- You can use color cues to catch and maintain their attention. Things like colorful notes around the house can remind them of tasks or appointments or anything relevant happening in their life.
- Make sure they have enough rest so that sleep deprivation won't worsen their apathy.

Wandering

This is a common behavior in patients with dementia. It can happen at any time of the day, although specific patients might be triggered by something in particular. For example, the patient might feel lost, looking for why they stood up in the first place, looking for something they think they lost, having hallucinations, or feeling the need to go home. Wandering around one's own house but thinking they are elsewhere is very common, simply because they don't recognize the objects around them. This is a very upsetting and frustrating circumstance for them, in which they feel unsafe and bewildered. Here are some tips for you to try with your patient.

- Remove the triggers that initiate the response. If your patient starts expressing the need to go home after seeing a coat or a hat, remove those objects from their sight.
- Promptly respond to their emotional triggers. For example, if you see them being very sad or upset, try to reassure them, letting them know they are safe at home with you. Try to distract them and get them interested in something they enjoy.
- Last but not least, in order to avoid unsafe situations where the patient leaves the house, try locking or disguising doors. If you add a door latch, try putting it at the top of the door and have it installed at a time when the patient does not see the installation. At some stages of dementia, dark-colored rugs help with wandering because some patients see the dark mat as a hole.

Obstinance

Stubbornness usually comes as a reaction when the patient doesn't understand the source of their frustration or the reasons for which they might be wrong. A good way to correct these reactions is to speak respectfully, use kind words, and have a lot of patience. When your patient struggles to understand something and exhibits the classic stubborn-like behavior, such as not responding to questions or requests to do something, take a minute to assess what you are asking. Make sure you give them the time needed to answer one question at a time. If they refuse to do a task you ask of them (bathing, going for a walk), realize that these things can be done later or another day and can be accomplished with a different approach. Sometimes, you'll experience obstinate behavior because they feel they don't have control over things. Losing their independence is difficult as it would be for anyone.

Take note of what is going on at the time of the obstinance in case there's a trigger causing the behavior. It's easier to keep a written log many times since you, the caregiver, are very likely exhausted most days and may not recall these things at a later time.

Agnosia

Not recognizing objects and faces is referred to as agnosia. It's a prevalent condition in dementia patients. It also refers to the inability to navigate familiar environments and can be one of the causes of typical wandering behavior.

"I once saw Mr. Brown hearing the phone ringing and going around the room looking for it. I realized he didn't recognize the phone, which was on the table next to where he'd been sitting."

When this kind of situation starts, you should teach your patient the basics of using objects the way you would with a child.

- Instead of being dramatic and letting them know their difficulties, try instead to direct their hands, eyes, and attention toward the object. If they can't see a fork, take it and put it in their hands; if they can't see a phone, lead them to the exact spot where the sound comes from.
- Take advantage of your patient's tendency to follow your behavior. If you catch their attention and show them how to sit on a chair, open a door, pick up a fork, they'll imitate you. You can use this to teach them things they've forgotten.
- Put colorful labels on things and objects. This will catch their attention and help them recognize certain items. A picture of a plate on the cabinet where the plates are and a photo with the person's name on it

are examples of how you can help your loved one recognize things.

- Whenever you instruct them verbally, do it in a simple and straightforward manner. This way, you will avoid confusing them and boost their confidence.

Apraxia

Another common condition that develops in dementia patients is called Apraxia, or the inability to perform motor tasks. Because of this, patients will have difficulties performing a task based on a verbal command, like dressing, eating, and bathing. This wide group of problems greatly challenges the patients' independence and the caregiver's ability to care for them. Here are some useful tips for managing such behaviors.

- Always make sure your patient is wearing comfortable clothes so it's easier for the patient to move.
- While helping them with verbal instructions, ensure things are in the correct order to help the patient use them. For clothes, the first layer would be underwear, then a shirt, and so on.
- When they have to carry out a simple task, make sure you eliminate any distractions from their surroundings (if the task is getting dressed, remove

any books, house keys, or anything that could interfere).

Bathing difficulties

Another very demanding activity dementia patients and caregivers are confronted with is bathing. It is a very delicate process in which the patient is literally exposed to you, and for this reason, they might feel ashamed and fragile. Because of possible perceptual hallucinations, they might also be afraid of water or the bathtub itself, which they might see as deep and threatening. In order to make this process as smooth as possible, it's important that you establish a relationship of mutual trust with your patient. Try applying the following tips to improve this experience and make it pleasant for both of you.

- Constantly involve your patient throughout the process. Ask them to hold shampoos or sponges for you, and even let them attempt to wash by themselves when possible. To make them feel less embarrassed, it's pivotal that you make them think that they're only being helped rather than completely assisted.
- Make sure the bathroom is warm even in the summertime. This can be accomplished by turning up the heat or turning on the hot water and letting the heat from the water warm the room. You can be

in the other room with your patient choosing clean clothes while the room is warming. When ready for them to undress, ask the patient if you can look at their feet. Asking like this will make them feel in control, and they'll likely say ok. Take their shoes and socks off for them. Ask if they need help undressing. Then, give the patient a washcloth when they enter the shower. You can use one and let them wash where they can. A shower head with a hose that stretches can be helpful here as well as a shower chair.

- For a tub bath, determine if they're more scared of an empty bathtub or a full one. If they're afraid of the water, let them get in the tub with a little water, then fill it. If, on the other hand, they're uncomfortable about entering an empty bathtub, fill it beforehand; Make sure you're careful that the water is at the right temperature.

- Try to prepare the bathroom before they enter. Place all the needed towels, soaps, and items you need within arm's reach so that you won't risk neglecting your patient, who could fall or get hurt.

Whether you are dealing with issues related to anger or perceptual difficulties, apathy, or aggressiveness, it's important that you apply the seven tips listed at the beginning of this chapter to help shape your patient's behavior according to specific circumstances. Observing and listening to your patient is always fundamental. Acknowledging their unique features and personality traits will make them feel comforted and loved.

7

DIET AND NUTRITION

WHY WON'T PEOPLE WITH DEMENTIA EAT OR DRINK?

A hallucination they're experiencing, the temperature of the food, the type of food you offer, not being able to see the food on their plate, or too many options to choose from are just some of the reasons a Dementia patient might stop eating or drinking. The disease might have altered their taste buds, and slightly spicier or sweeter food might have become a disliked flavor for them. When planning their meal routine, consult them about what they like and don't. If you force them to eat at a time of the day they are not used to, they might refuse—ignoring their difficulties and thinking that they'll eat when hungry might also be very detrimental to them. They may forget to eat, and this could lead to weight loss and other physical difficulties because you think they're just not hungry. You can add vitamin supplements into shakes and puddings and make all meals finger foods to help keep them nourished. As the disease progresses, your patient may refuse to eat to the point that you may have to give them fewer healthy options just to get them to eat. Make sure to give your loved one plenty of time to eat. An hour or more may become the length of time it takes for them to eat. Keep in mind your patient has no control over this behavior, so plan for this extra time for them to eat. The doctor can also prescribe medication to increase the appetite, which should be considered if your loved one is losing too much weight.

Keep Hydrated

Hydration is a fundamental characteristic of every living organism. We all need water to survive. As we get older, however, thirst becomes less evident as a feeling and our body loses its capacity to store water as much water as before. The lack of feeling thirsty in addition to not retaining as much water can result in drinking less and lead to dehydration. This is the reason why older people are encouraged to drink a certain amount of liquids even if they don't feel the need for it. In dementia patients, this weaker sensitivity for thirst is even more pronounced, and a caregiver needs to be careful that this doesn't transform into dehydration.

Among the main reasons why dementia patients don't feel thirst anymore is that the brain part responsible for regulating this bodily function is compromised, but there are other causes. The already attenuated thirst feeling might be exacerbated by forgetting: in fact, they might not remember the last time they drank, as well as where to get water from, where the glasses are, and so on. If the patient also suffers from speech difficulties, it will be very hard for them to communicate the need to drink to you. Furthermore, other existing medical conditions and medications can worsen dehydration. For example, diabetes can cause rapid fluid loss, while some medications prescribed to Alzheimer's patients can increase urination. Also, frequent illnesses to which dementia patients are more exposed might make drinking and eating more uncomfortable. When looking for signs of dehydration, if you're unsure whether your patient is drinking too much or too little, you should observe any change in their usual behaviors and any signs of fatigue, muscle cramping, or headaches. You could also look at whether the urine is dark/amber-colored and whether it has a strong smell because this could be a sign of dehydration.

Let's go through some useful tips to combat dehydration.

- Encourage your patient to drink without forcing them. You can do this by entertaining them in a conversation and casually drinking water. Your patient will likely copy what you're doing.

- Keep water close to them. Set drinking reminders for yourself to make sure they drink. There are a variety of different products you can purchase to help your patient remember to drink. For example, online, you can find water bottles that light up every hour, which, if kept close to your patient, might help.
- Make drinking pleasurable for them. You can do this by adding blueberries, cucumbers, cherries, or anything they like to the water. The bright colors might also catch their attention and encourage them to look for water by themselves.
- Hydration doesn't only come directly from water; there are a variety of foods that are highly hydrating. For example, watermelon, cucumber, yogurts, and broths have rich water content and can be added to your patient's diet. Homemade popsicles made with fruit juice can help with increasing fluid intake without all the sugar of store-bought ones.

Eating Habit & Taste Changes

Although knowing what your patient's favorite foods are might help you in some instances, many patients completely lose interest in foods they enjoyed before and prefer others instead. This can happen because their taste buds have changed. After all, they've forgotten what they liked before. Another reason may be because they see you eating something different, and they want to copy your behavior. When and if this occurs, you should accommodate their preferences.

If they start asking for more flavored options, you can try bolder dishes adding flavors like curry, soy sauce seasoning, saffron, and ginger. When experimenting with different foods, you should always keep in mind your patient's allergies and physiological characteristics. For example, if they have problems with constipation, opt for a fiber-rich diet, or if they have the opposite problem, you should try serving them binding foods such as boiled potatoes, crackers, applesauce, peanut butter, etc.

Managing their food intake also means being extremely careful about what they ingest, which might sometimes be things other than food. As the disease progresses, some patients might struggle to recognize certain objects and mistake them for food, especially when hungry. In order to avoid this, try emptying the table of any item other than food, and make sure harmful substances like coins, soaps, cleaning agents, and the like are not accessible to your patient.

GETTING THE RIGHT NUTRITION

As previously mentioned, the right diet for your patient has to be based on their taste preferences but should also consist of healthy food. Generally speaking, there are a few rules that should always be remembered when preparing a meal.

The amount of food they eat should be proportional to their weight. It's important not to provide too much or too little food. The patient's diet should always be balanced, containing a little bit of every type of nutrient including proteins, carbohydrates, fibers, vitamins, minerals, and water. At the same time, if your patient is a senior, there are a few foods you should avoid altogether, which are not generally recommended for older people, regardless of them having dementia or not. Here are some things to avoid when preparing meals for your loved one.

1. Raw or undercooked foods such as eggs and meat
2. Fast foods, such as french fries, doughnuts, and burgers, can be very detrimental to your patient's health. This is because they are very caloric but empty of needed nutrients, filling your patient's stomach and preventing them from eating healthy foods.
3. Margarine - researchers have found that diacetyl, which is an ingredient in margarine, may cause protein clusters to form in the brain.
4. Grapefruit is not the best option if your patient is taking medications for high blood pressure, insomnia, or anxiety. This fruit has the potential to increase the level of certain medications in the blood. This higher level of drug in the system can increase the side effects.
5. Avoid too much salt and too much sugar.

6. Limit saturated fats because some of these fats may increase some symptoms related to dementia.

7. Avoid MSG (monosodium glutamate), which is a flavor enhancer. This seasoning can cause an exacerbation of symptoms in dementia patients. While this is an additive you'll find in many restaurants and take-out foods, you should also check ingredient labels in many frozen dinners and other foods.

8. Avoid processed foods and meats.

Just as there are some foods to avoid, there are also some foods that are particularly good for those with dementia. Let's go over some nutritious options for your patient.

Best Foods for Dementia Patients

Some foods are thought to slow down cognitive decline and are specifically beneficial for dementia patients. Vegetables and legumes are essential to sustain memory function. This is because they equip the brain with important vitamins, like B6, that support mood, sleep, and appetite. Vitamin B6 can be found in various plant and animal foods, such as tuna, salmon, and chickpeas.

Other simple vegetables that support brain functions are green vegetables, such as spinach, broccoli, and cabbage, which are rich in vitamin E, calcium, and manganese.

If your patient is a fan of sweet foods, on the other hand, there is nothing better to eat than fruits. Blueberries, in particular, were shown to improve brain function and slow down neurodegeneration (Krikorian et al., 2010). These fruits also reduce the risk of developing cardiovascular diseases by lowering blood cholesterol and enhancing the function and health of the arteries. Your patient should eat "many colors of the rainbow," meaning that there are fruits of other colors that can benefit their cognitive health as well. Oranges and apricots, for example, are a great source of potassium, pineapples of manganese, and kiwis of vitamin C.

If they are fond of sweet tastes, they will surely love cocoa, which has anti-inflammatory and antioxidant properties. Cocoa, in fact, reduces the risks of inflammation while improving heart health and cholesterol levels. However, when cocoa is processed into chocolate, it loses some of its health benefits. To avoid that, there are other ways in which cocoa can be consumed.

- Add a spoonful of cocoa powder to your patient's favorite yogurt (you may have to add a little water to the cocoa powder to dissolve first) or stir some in their morning coffee.
- Add some cocoa nibs (cracked cocoa beans, dried and fermented) to salads, smoothies, ice cream, or oatmeal. One tablespoon of nibs contains about 2 grams of fiber and has antioxidants. These can be found at most grocery stores or online.

Fish is another important source of different fundamental vitamins for a healthy lifestyle. It contains vitamin A, which improves tissue health, vitamin B3 for overall brain health, vitamin B6, which is fundamental for mood regulation, sleep, and appetite, vitamin B12 for nerve cell protection, and vitamin D, which regulates calcium and phosphorus levels in the blood.

There are some specific foods that help regulate gut bacteria and promote tryptophan absorption, which is an amino acid that allows the production of serotonin and melatonin. These foods include yogurt, cottage cheese, kefir, sauerkraut, and Kombucha. Kombucha is a popular drink in the US and worldwide and is made of beneficial bacteria. It's a long-fermented drink made of sugary tea and a culture of yeasts called SCOBY. Its taste is slightly acidic and fizzy, making it very similar to lemonade, prosecco, or apple cider.

Practical Tips To Help Them Eat More

1. Make sure there is a contrast in the color of the plate and the food. If food is too similar to the color of the plate, your loved one may not be able to see the food. Studies have found that dementia patients eat approximately 25% more when their food is on a red, blue, or yellow plate versus a white one. Use patterned tablecloths or placemats sparingly, as this could be distracting and confusing to your patient.

Stick with solid colors that are different from the plate color.

2. Try putting smaller quantities of food on the plate. Arrange each food so that it's right next to or touching the other.

3. Get them to mirror your actions. They may not know how or what to do and will likely copy what you are doing if you are sitting directly across from them. Make eye contact, smile, and make a big deal of how good the food tastes. This may take some patience and make mealtimes much longer.

4. While you do want to praise the food, make sure you don't talk much. You want your patient to eat, and for dementia patients, it can be confusing to do more than one thing at a time.

5. Try putting foods they've always liked on the plate but realize that you may need to try different textures of foods or completely different foods due to a change in their taste buds. Sometimes a food they once loved may now smell bad to them. Remember, they're not trying to upset you by not eating foods they've always eaten, this is the disease.

6. Cut food into smaller, bite-size pieces and make sure the food is not too hot or too cold.

7. Have small portions of "finger foods" available throughout the day rather than just three typical meals per day. Utilizing finger foods helps with the challenges later on in the disease when difficulty

with holding and using utensils is experienced. See the quick reference guide listed next for some examples.

FINGER FOODS FOR DEMENTIA PATIENTS

- Tuna salad sandwich strips
- Chicken salad sandwich strips
- Egg salad sandwich strips
- Try putting the above in leafy greens (lettuce wraps)
- Salmon patties
- Sardines (on a plate - they may cut themselves on the can)
- Fish Sticks
- Meatloaf Fingers
- Meatballs
- Mini Quesadillas
- Chicken Nuggets
- Shrimp Cocktail
- Edamame
- Nuts
- Peanut Butter and Jelly
- Pimento Cheese Sandwiches
- Egg Omelet strips
- Peanut butter on a plastic spoon
- Crepes
- Breakfast muffins
- Biscuit Pieces

- Croissant
- Mini bagels
- Biscuit Halves
- Egg Bread/French Toast Fingers
- Tofu sticks
- Silver Dollar Pancakes
- Waffle Sticks
- Room temperature oatmeal
- Ravioli with or without sauce to dip it in (refrigerated aisle of the grocery store)
- Sweet Potato Fries
- Boiled new potatoes halved
- Mini Quiches
- Cheese Cubes/Sticks
- Soft cheese cubes
- Mashed potatoes
- Tater tots
- Broccoli, cauliflower, tomatoes
- Avocado Pieces
- Hummus
- Peaches
- Blueberries
- Raspberries
- Watermelon
- Mandarin Orange/tangerine pieces
- Bananas
- Pears
- Cantelope

- Nectarines
- Strawberries
- Jello Pieces - (Made with less water to be firmer than the regular recipe)
- Pound cake pieces
- Angel food pieces
- Graham crackers
- Shakes/Smoothies with protein powder and nutrition supplements
- Yogurt cups or bars
- Granola Bars
- Pudding cups (like snack pack) room temp

Now that you're familiar with the difficulties you'll be facing with eating, drinking, and nutrition, you'll be able to plan ahead and use the tips provided to overcome some of the frustrating parts of being a caregiver. You'll worry about your patient when they don't eat or drink as they did, but you now have the tools to provide as much help as possible. This part of the journey is often challenging, but you can do this! Next, we'll talk about some myths surrounding dementia and some other advice for you, the caregiver.

8

MYTHS & OTHER ADVICE

COMMON MYTHS ABOUT DEMENTIA

- **Memory loss always indicates dementia.**

There are many reasons for forgetfulness and memory loss, such as depression, side effects from medication, infections, and other health issues.

- **Everyone gets dementia when they are older.**

According to a report by the Alzheimer's Association, Dementia is not an inevitable part of aging.

- **Alzheimer's and dementia are the same thing**.

There are many different types of dementia, and Alzheimer's is one of those types.

- **Dementia only affects older people.**

Early onset dementia can affect younger people Ages 30 - 64

- **Dementia is hereditary.**

While the chances of having dementia may be higher within families, it does not mean that all relatives will develop dementia.

- **You can prevent dementia.**

There are things you can do to decrease your risk of developing dementia and things to do to delay the onset of the disease; however, there is no proven way to prevent dementia. There's also no evidence to suggest that any vitamin regimen will prevent dementia.

WHAT NOT TO SAY TO SOMEONE WITH DEMENTIA - WHAT TO SAY INSTEAD

- Don't remind them that a loved one is dead. If they don't remember, you may cause them to live through the grief of the loss again. Change the subject.
- Don't argue with the dementia patient or tell them they are wrong. Change the subject.
- Don't say, "do you remember," instead, say, "I remember."
- Don't say "I just told you,'" Instead, repeat what you said in exactly the same words. They simply may not remember.
- Don't correct them if they say something that is wrong or have a different memory of something that happened. Just continue with the conversation.
- Instead of asking open-ended questions, ask specific questions that the patient can answer yes, or no to.
- Don't speak about them to others as if they're not there or don't understand. Instead of saying that their dementia is getting worse, go into another room to discuss a topic such as this with the other person.
- Don't bring up subjects that upset them. Keep things on a positive note.
- Don't ask them if they remember you. Tell them if they ask or say something to them, including your name.

- Don't ask, "what did you do this morning?" (They may not remember) Say "good morning," or "good morning," "I'm glad to see you, "it's a beautiful day," or something else positive.
- If they say, "you're not my son," don't say, yes, I am; say, "he'll be here later. Would you like to take a walk?"

HELPING CHILDREN UNDERSTAND

Children who have family members with dementia will likely ask questions when they notice something is different. They may ask questions like, "why doesn't Mimi ever want to play with me anymore?" "Why did grandpa get angry when I was playing in the living room?" " What's wrong with Uncle Jimmy?" He acted like he doesn't know who I am. It's best to answer these questions honestly.

Make sure you explain in language that is age appropriate and, whenever possible, give children help with suggestions on what to do instead. Enlist their help with the patient. Make sure you let them know that laughing at their loved one may hurt the loved one's feelings. Listen to your children, and make sure you answer all of their questions. This may be a scary time for them as well. Keep things upbeat and let them know that the dementia patient still loves them. Suggest things for them to do with their loved one. "Why don't you take your dolls and play with them with Mimi." "Maybe you could take a walk with Grandpa in the backyard." Why don't you get the picture album of our vacation and look at some pictures with Uncle Jimmy?" or "This weekend, we'll work on a memory box with Mimi." There are many children's books online and in the library specifically for helping children understand dementia.

FOLLOWING A ROUTINE

One of the most important things from the very beginning of the dementia diagnosis is following a routine. There are many reasons this will benefit you and the patient. Short-term memory loss is usually one of the first things dementia patients experience, but our routines are stored in our long-term memory. Having established ways from the beginning will help your loved one feel more independent and in control, and this may help well into the middle stages of the disease. Not being able to remember recent events or how to do simple tasks can be quite frustrating for your loved one. Following a daily ritual can help them continue to do many things and make them feel independent in a world that has now made them more dependent on others. This can decrease anxiety and help your loved one cope with some of the changes that are happening.

A routine also helps you, the caregiver, know what to expect and will make it easier to plan your schedule around your needs and duties in other aspects of your life. When establishing a routine, one thing to be aware of is your loved one's previous habits. They likely have a precise manner in which they do things already, and it's best if you try to incorporate as many of those things into the regimen now. Additional changes at this point may be upsetting to your loved one and may be a challenge due to their short-term memory loss. However, there'll be times when you can't keep to the routines due to circumstances beyond your control. You'll need to be somewhat flexible during these times and realize that your goal is to provide some stabilization for your patient and yourself so just do your best.

One final note about establishing routines, whenever possible, incorporate music and physical activity and allow your loved one to help with as much as possible around the house. You must also think about organizing the schedule so that it will allow you to take a break some days for a couple of hours at a time and take time out for others in your family. Planning time for yourself and adding it to the day-to-day tasks early on will make some things less stressful in the future. In the next chapter, we'll address your future and discuss how to take care of yourself.

PART III

YOU AND YOUR FUTURE

"Like airplane passengers, let's not forget to put on our own oxygen masks first ... we are no good to our loved ones if we collapse under the strain."

— PETER B.

9

YOUR WELL-BEING MATTERS TOO

In this chapter, I want to remind you that you are now the caregiver for *two* people: your loved one *and* yourself. We'll go over tips and advice on how to maintain your physical and mental well-being while at the same time caring for your loved one and juggling all the demands that are expected of you. We'll also go over why allowing others to help you is so important. At the end of this book, we've listed resources for you to find help when you need it. You are not alone.

From the very moment you heard the diagnosis, you likely experienced anxiety, worry, grief, sadness, and anger. These are all normal feelings, but you can also still experience happiness, joy, and calmness. There are times on this journey when you'll need to put yourself and your health first. In putting yourself first, you may feel like you're being selfish and have feelings of guilt, experience loneliness, and, surprisingly, joy in being free, if only for a few hours. These feelings are normal.

Your physical and mental health will be challenged with the journey ahead, so putting yourself first at times in order to be able to care for your loved one will be vitally important. According to a June 2021 CDC report, parent caregivers that were filling both parenting and guardian/adult caregiver roles are 12 times more likely to have serious mental health symptoms, including suicidal thoughts. In fact, a CDC survey taken during the pandemic confirmed that as much as 70 percent of caregivers who were taking care of loved ones have anxiety, depression, or at least one other mental health issue. Another study finds that this mental health issue is magnified in Hispanic, Latino, or Black caregivers. Let's start with some basics for your mental health.

YOUR MENTAL HEALTH

As the disease progresses, you may find that you're required to be with the patient more frequently. You may be trying to work and raise children while spending more time taking care of your loved one with dementia. If not, you may now be limited with social contacts that you may have had previously due to not being able to leave your loved one at home alone. You'll need respite many times throughout this journey.

Respite - the Oxford Dictionary definition of this word is "a short period of rest or relief from something difficult or unpleasant."

You cannot let your loved one's illness take center stage. You'll likely have many other responsibilities when this diagnosis is made, and you must understand that taking care of your own physical and mental health is imperative.

Get out of the house and away from your loved one. Having someone sit even for an hour while you get a manicure, a pedicure, have coffee, have lunch or walk around a store you enjoy will be a great stress reliever and can improve your overall mental health. You may have to enlist family members, friends, and others to sit with your loved one while you take a break. One of the hardest things for most of us is to ask for help. It seems we feel like we're "bothering" others or admitting defeat if we ask for help, but this is not true.

You need someone who understands what you're going through. This could be a close friend that you can call or have coffee or lunch with once a week or once every other week. Sounding off on someone else sometimes helps us release pent-up feelings and puts us in a better mindset. Writing in a journal expressing your emotions can help too. If you feel embarrassed about your anger or dream that you could escape caring for your loved one, writing your feelings down may help with the frustrations these thoughts bring while allowing you to keep these feelings private.

Support groups, both online and in person, are the place to find others who have or are going through a similar journey. Support group members may have suggestions and ideas you haven't thought of. If you're going to an in-person group, it may or may not be helpful to take your loved one with you. No matter what, a support group will be an important part of this journey. Whether you build a team of individuals who are close to you or choose to choose others that are online and in other in-person groups, the benefit will be beyond what you may realize right now.

Don't isolate yourself. You must keep in contact with social connections and continue nurturing your relationships. Caring for your loved one can be lonely, and many caregivers tend to stop communicating with friends and family members due to the stress and exhaustion of the situation. You must stay connected to these lifelines.

YOUR PHYSICAL HEALTH

Make sure you're eating healthy and drinking plenty of water. You'll likely have more demands physically, and you'll need to be fueled and rested with the additional responsibilities you've taken on.

Exercise helps relieve stress, gives you more energy, and helps with sleep. Make sure you're getting some type of exercise daily. This could be a brisk walk around the yard, dancing in the living room, or any other exercise that increases your heart rate. You can exercise while your loved one watches or while they are occupied with something else. If they're watching, know that they may try to mirror what you're doing and will get exercise too. Try to get at least 30 minutes three times a week, but even 15 minutes of exercise several times a week can help.

Make sure you attend to your own physical health. Going to the dentist and your physician regularly is critical. Talk to your physician about any health concerns you have and inform them of your situation. They may be able to help identify stress symptoms you are unaware of and suggest ideas to help as well.

It's ok to laugh. Laughter releases endorphins and can increase circulation, help you relax, and improve your overall mood. Watching a funny movie or a comedy show will be helpful for you and your loved one.

Get enough sleep. Caregivers often neglect to ensure they have a good night's sleep. During the day, limit caffeine and try not to take naps. A regular schedule for bedtime and waking up is essential as well, even on your days off.

If you've been trying to go to sleep for 20 minutes and can't, you should get out of bed and try reading or doing something relaxing and then try again. Try the 4-7-8 method. Although this does not work for everyone, the technique is aimed at reducing your anxiety. Here's how to do it: take a deep breath in through your nose for 4 seconds, hold it for 7 seconds, then exhale through your mouth (with force) for 8 seconds. Repeat four times. As a side note, this is a good exercise when you are frustrated as well. Do the same technique and repeat twice. ***You may feel light-headed when you first start doing this, so make sure you are sitting or lying down before starting this technique****

If you can't hold your breath as long as specified above, try the same technique: inhaling for 2 seconds, holding your breath for 3.5 seconds, and then exhaling for 4 seconds.

The future ahead may not be easy, but taking care of yourself and not getting "lost" in the disease will help with the challenges you'll face. Making sure you are well physically and mentally and keeping your own identity will allow you to care for your patient better and may help you find a way to make the most of your time with them. Next, we'll discuss some decisions that need to be addressed and resources for additional information.

10

LONG-TERM CARE AND END-OF-LIFE DECISIONS

As unpleasant as it will be to discuss, there are some specific things that must be planned and accomplished after you receive a diagnosis of dementia. We'll talk about some potential long-term care options, but first, we'll begin with some hard decisions that should be made early on if possible. Planning and discussing the end of life at the beginning of the diagnosis may allow your loved one to participate in these tough decisions so now is the time to talk about their end of life wishes. There is no way to determine how quickly a person's dementia will progress. Some people with dementia will need support very soon after their diagnosis. In contrast, others will stay independent for several years. Dementia doesn't follow an exact or specific set of steps that happen in the same way for every person with dementia. So, while the end of life is likely many years away, don't assume that you know what their wishes are.

As we discuss different topics, be aware that what we go over should still be addressed now, even if your loved one cannot participate in the decision-making process. I assure you that planning now and knowing what steps to take later will provide some relief to you when you get to this stage in the disease process. Feeding tubes, respirators, IV hydration, CPR, and Hospice are some of the things to be discussed. You should understand that refusing or withdrawing treatment is letting the disease take its course and is not suicide.

A living will should be prepared for the dementia patient. A living will is the written instructions of what the patient wants if they're unable to communicate their wishes (or not considered competent to make those decisions).

A durable power of attorney for healthcare should be prepared. This document will name a specific person to make health care decisions in case the patient cannot. This form is available at most hospitals and some office supply stores and is available to download for free online.

A durable power of attorney for finances is a form that specifies someone to make financial decisions for the patient.

A do not resuscitate order **(DNR)** should be discussed with the patient's physician. The DNR is an order signed by a doctor based on the patient's wishes. The DNR tells a medical team (such as paramedics) not to perform life-saving procedures *to restart the heart or breathing once they have ceased.* If your patient is in the hospital or at home and having trouble breathing, they would still receive all methods to alleviate and correct this condition. The key thing to remember when discussing a DNR is the fact that the order deals with *what to do if the heart or breathing has ceased.* If the heart or breathing has stopped, *CPR would not be performed* if the patient has a DNR. If emergency personnel arrive at the home, you will need to let them know the patient has a DNR, and in most cases, they'll need to see a copy.

For this reason, many patients keep the DNR on the refrigerator or in a folder easily located if emergency personnel are called.

Other planning should include making sure that you agree on how your loved one would like to have their finances handled. This includes having a joint owner on an account and specifying how the dementia patient will be able to access their funds. Beneficiaries named on policies and monetary accounts also need to be reviewed and updated if necessary.

A copy of these documents should be provided to doctors, family members, and other healthcare providers, such as hospice and home health providers.

Finally, any necessary passwords for accounts that the caregiver will need to access should be recorded and put in a safe place.

How do you know if it's time for memory care or a different living situation?

HERE ARE 7 SIGNS IT'S TIME TO STOP CARING FOR YOUR LOVED ONE AT HOME

1. If your loved one is constantly wandering off and the methods you have in place are not keeping them at home, they may leave and become lost. When your loved one leaves home and wanders, they may have a fall or walk in front of a car or other dangerous situations.

2. Aggressive behavior is another indicator that your loved one may not be appropriate to stay home. Behaviors such as irritability, agitation, and sundowning can worsen as the disease progresses. Sometimes, these aggressive behaviors can put you and your loved one at risk.

3. As the patient gets to later stages, they may have chronic incontinence. If you're having difficulty getting the patient to the toilet or lifting or helping the patient, this is a sign that your loved one may no longer be safe at home. Chronic incontinence can lead to infections. Difficulty in helping the patient

move around the home could put the caregiver at risk if they fall with the patient or try to "catch" the patient.

4. When your loved one can no longer walk or has difficulty getting around and is limited to a chair most of the day, they may no longer be appropriate to care for at home.

5. If your loved one's hallucinations worsen, this could be dangerous for you. When they see things that are not there and honestly believe what they see is real, they may act in ways they never would before the deterioration of their brain.

6. Refusing to let you help may be another indicator that the patient is not appropriate for home care any longer. When the patient refuses to eat, refuses to let you help them clean up after an incontinence episode, or acts out in other ways refusing your help, their overall health and yours could be in jeopardy.

7. Your loved one may no longer be appropriate to care for at home if you have caregiver burnout. Often, caregivers have put off taking care of their own health needs and can no longer care for their loved one at home 24/7.

Here are some things to consider when looking for a care facility for your loved one.

More often than not, the cost of a facility will be a determining factor in where you'll be able to place your loved one.

Some facilities are designed or have areas specifically for dementia patients. Most of these facilities are secured, so the patient does not wander off. When looking for a care facility, you should visit quite a few. You can make appointments to discuss services and pricing, but you should also show up without an appointment at several different times (especially when you narrow your choices down). You'll want to notice if the facility looks clean and whether or not there are any unpleasant odors. Talk with the staff and other patients' family members you see visiting. In the US, ask to see the facility's state survey inspection report. Ask for a copy of the CQC (Care Quality Commission) report in the UK. Information can also be found online for the US and the UK.

When you visit facilities, choose different times of the day and make sure you go at mealtime and observe the food that is being served to residents. Here are some questions to ask.

1. How does the facility ensure nutritious meals, and what do they do about specific dietary requirements?
2. Can the family join the patient for dinner?
3. Look at the residents to see if they look clean and if their clothes are clean.
4. How does the facility communicate any health or other issues to the family?
5. Does the staff contact family members when planning or changing care plans?
6. What specific medical and personal care is provided?
7. Is laundry service provided?

8. Are pets allowed?
9. Is there a barber or beautician that comes to the facility?
10. What is the ratio of nurses to patients, and is there a registered nurse on the premises at all times?
11. How often is a physician there, and how often will they see your loved one?
12. Is the staff trained in behavioral issues, and what techniques do they use?
13. Does the facility take residents to medical appointments if they're not being seen by a doctor who visits the facility?
14. How does the facility handle E/R visits? Do they send a representative with the patient if emergency services are called?
15. What is the discharge policy?
16. Does the facility provide end-of-life care and allow hospice to see patients?
17. What situation would prompt the facility to discharge the patient, and how much notice would you receive?

In the US, traditional Medicare will pay one hundred percent for the first 20 days a patient is in a skilled nursing facility to receive rehab services. After that, for days 21 - 100, the patient is responsible for a portion of the costs (usually 20%). After 100 days, Medicare does not pay for skilled nursing. This means most families pay out of pocket for long-term care. A recent survey (Genworth, 2021) shows that the national average cost of long-term care for a private room in a skilled nursing facility is $9,034. For a semi-private room, the average cost is $7,908. In some states in the US, Medicaid will pay for long-term care, but there are specific rules related to income and assets. Each situation is unique, so it's best to consult an Elder Care attorney to get advice on navigating the requirement. Elder care attorneys listen to each situation and give advice on what is best for your situation. They specialize in preserving and transferring assets to help a spouse avoid poverty when their loved one enters a nursing facility.

HOSPICE CARE: WHEN IS IT TIME?

Hospice care is end-of-life care to make patients more comfortable during the last months of life. There are many benefits to hospice care, but sadly, even though Medicare and some insurances pay 100% for hospice, many families are not aware of or do not want to have hospice help. Some of the items they provide are incontinence supplies, bed pads, hospital beds, respite care while caregivers take a break or go out of town for family events, volunteers to come to sit with the patient, and many other things.

Hospice can be initiated when there is the expectation that the patient has six months or less to live. Unfortunately, this can make determining when a dementia patient is Hospice appropriate very difficult since there's no way to estimate the remaining time a dementia patient has. There are two criteria that can be used for dementia patients to determine if they are eligible for Hospice.

One is the Reisberg Functional Assessment Staging (FAST scale). On this scale, the patient must rank stage seven. At stage seven on the FAST scale, they are unable to do things such as bathe or walk without assistance, speak less than six words a day, and are usually unable to smile.

The second is that they must also have an additional comorbidity. Comorbidities are additional illnesses such as COPD, CHF, cancer, and congenital heart disease. A diagnosis of pneumonia or sepsis or frequent E/R visits are also qualifying factors.

Hospice is available to the patient even if they are in a facility. As well as providing nursing services for the patient to keep them comfortable, there are other benefits at no cost for the family of the patient during care and after the patient is gone. These benefits include grief counselling, a medical social worker to help navigate end-of-life issues such as funeral and burial services, and bereavement support groups.

"Life is a circle. The end of one journey is the beginning of the next."

— JOSEPH M. MARSHALL III

My intention with this book was to provide you with enough resilience and knowledge to face the journey of caring for an individual affected by dementia. I also celebrate your bravery and courage to approach this read in the first place.

If you enjoyed this book and found it helpful, please leave a review on Amazon so that others may find it too.

Scan below to leave a quick review!

https://geni.us/Jhtnr

CONCLUSION

Dementia is a terrible disease and being the caregiver of a dementia patient is heart-wrenching. As researchers try to find a cure, know that none of this happened due to anything you or your loved one did or didn't do. You've learned about seven types of dementia and now have problem-solving strategies to manage this journey. You have the tools and knowledge to provide the best care for your loved one (and yourself!) as they go through the stages of dementia. You and your loved one still have many beautiful memories to make, so let that be of comfort to you.

"There will come a time when your loved one is gone, and you will find comfort in the fact that you were their caregiver."

— **KAREN COETZER**

US RESOURCES FOR THE CAREGIVER

Centers for Disease Control and Prevention
https://www.cdc.gov/aging/aginginfo/alzheimers.htm

Dementia Society of America
https://www.cdc.gov/aging/aginginfo/alzheimers.htm

Lewy Body Dementia Association
https://www.lbda.org/

Support for Vets with Dementia
https://www.va.gov/GERIATRICS/pages/
Alzheimers_and_Dementia_Care.asp

National Aphasia Association
https://www.aphasia.org/aphasia-resources/dementia/?gclid=Cj0KC
QiAyMKbBhD1ARIsANs7rEGZxmONfHyquAsJSCKgs-qCyz64hOYSJH
POdfrt6-YJdgvGP1RQW3waAu6yEALw_wcB

Center Watch - Clinical Trials
https://www.centerwatch.com/directories/1068-useful-resources/list-
ing/2641-dementia-society-of-America

Parkinson and Movement Disorder Alliance
https://www.pmdalliance.org/

For People with Parkinsons
https://www.jaxhopeinc.org/

Michael J Fox Foundation for Parkinson's Research
https://www.michaeljfox.org/

Parkinson's Foundation
https://www.parkinson.org/

International Parkinson and Movement Disorder Society
https://www.movementdisorders.org/MDS/Resources/Patient-Education.htm

Memory Cafe Directory
https://www.memorycafedirectory.com/
Dementia Friendly America
https://www.dfamerica.org/

Centers for Medicare and Medicaid Services
https://www.cms.gov/

Compare Nursing Home and Health Providers
https://www.medicare.gov/care-compare/

Alzheimer's Association
https://www.alz.org/

Resources from federal government agencies for people with
Alzheimer's disease and related dementias
https://www.alzheimers.gov/

Alzheimer's Foundation
https://alzfdn.org/

UK RESOURCES FOR THE CAREGIVER

Dementia Support in the UK
https://www.nhs.uk/conditions/dementia/help-and-support/

Care Quality Commision - Independent Regulator of Health and Social Care in England
https://www.cqc.org.uk/

Dementia Nurse Charity
https://www.dementiauk.org/

UK Advice Line
https://www.ageuk.org.uk/services/in-your-area/dementia-support/

Young Dementia Network
https://www.youngdementianetwork.org/

Guideposts Trust
https://guideposts.org.uk/

Lewy Body Society
https://www.lewybody.org/contact-us/

Rare Dementia Support
https://www.raredementiasupport.org/

Hope Again Bereavement Support
https://www.hopeagain.org.uk/

Inspire - Northern Ireland
https://www.inspirewellbeing.org/

Alzheimer Scotland
https://www.alzscot.org/

Alzheimer's Society
https://www.alzheimers.org.uk/

Aged Care Homes in Australia
https://www.myagedcare.gov.au/aged-care-homes

REFERENCES

Oxford Languages and Google - English | Oxford Languages. (2022b, August 12). https://languages.oup.com/google-dictionary-en/

Memory, Forgetfulness, and Aging: What's Normal and What's Not? (n.d.). National Institute on Aging. https://www.nia.nih.gov/health/memory-forgetfulness-and-aging-whats-normal-and-whats-not

Vascular Dementia: Causes, Symptoms, and Treatments. (n.d.). National Institute on Aging. https://www.nia.nih.gov/health/vascular-dementia

Aducanumab Approved for Treatment of Alzheimerâs Disease. (n.d.). Alzheimer's Disease and Dementia. https://www.alz.org/alzheimers-dementia/treatments/aducanumab

biopharma-reporter.com. (2021, July 29). *Prothena's monoclonal antibody and vaccine show promise in AD treatment and prevention.* https://www.biopharma-reporter.com/Article/2021/07/29/Prothena-s-monoclonal-antibody-and-vaccine-show-promise-in-AD-treatment-and-prevention

Statistics. (n.d.). Parkinson's Foundation. https://www.parkinson.org/understanding-parkinsons/statistics

Fernandes, C. (2022, October 14). *What Is Lewy Body Dementia?* Lewy Body Dementia Association. https://www.lbda.org/what-is-lbd/

Deep brain stimulation (DBS) for the treatment of Parkinson's disease and other movement disorders | National Institute of Neurological Disorders and Stroke. (n.d.). https://www.ninds.nih.gov/about-ninds/impact/ninds-contributions-approved-therapies/deep-brain-stimulation-dbs-treatment-parkinsons-disease-and-other-movement-disorders

Global Prevalence of Young-Onset Dementia: A Systematic Review and Meta-analysis. (2021, September 21). https://pubmed.ncbi.nlm.nih.gov. https://pubmed.ncbi.nlm.nih.gov/34279544/

(2022), 2022 Alzheimer's disease facts and figures. Alzheimer's Dement., 18: 700-789. https://doi.org/10.1002/alz.12638

https://www.prb.org/resources/fact-sheet-u-s-dementia-trends/ . (n.d.)

Satery, J. (2020, February 14). *5 Foods Older Adults with Dementia Should Avoid.*

Home Care Assistance of Arlington. https://www.homecareassistancear lingtontx.com/foods-for-elderly-people-to-avoid-if-they-have-dementia/

Spelman, K. (2018, December 6). *Herbal Medicine for Alzheimer's Disease: Lion's Mane (Hericium erinaceus)*. Restorative Medicine. https://restorativemedi cine.org/journal/neurological-activity-lions-mane-hericium-erinaceus/? utm_source=ojs

Wilson, R. (2022, October 15). *10 Best Colored Plates for Dementia Patients*. AlzheimersLab. https://www.alzheimerslab.com/colored-plates-for-dementia-patients/

Newman, T. (2020, September 21). *Medical myths: All about dementia*. https://www.medicalnewstoday.com/articles/medical-myths-all-about-dementia

Alzheimer's Association. (2019). *2019 ALZHEIMER'S DISEASE FACTS AND FIGURES*. https://www.alz.org/. https://www.alz.org/media/documents/alzheimers-facts-and-figures-2019-r.pdf

Helping children understand dementia. (n.d.). Alzheimer Society of Canada. https://alzheimer.ca/en/help-support/i-have-friend-or-family-member-who-lives-dementia/helping-children-understand-dementia

Hitt, R. (2022, January 12). *Importance of Routine for Dementia | Where You Live Matters*. ASHA. https://www.whereyoulivematters.org/importance-of-routines-for-dementia/

Attention Required! | Cloudflare. (n.d.). https://memory.ucsf.edu/caregiving-support/caregiver-well-being

Rothschild, P. (2022, August 5). *Supporting unpaid caregivers in crisis: A talk with Alexandra Drane*. McKinsey & Company. https://www.mckinsey.com/industries/healthcare-systems-and-services/our-insights/supporting-unpaid-caregivers-in-crisis-a-talk-with-alexandra-drane

Mental health among parents of children aged <18 years and unpaid care-givers of adults during the COVID-19 pandemic – United States, December 2020 and February–March 2021, Centers for Disease Control and Prevention, June 18, 2021, cdc.gov. https://www.cdc.gov/mmwr/volumes/69/wr/mm6932a1.htm

Czeisler MÉ, Drane A, Winnay SS, Capodilupo ER, Czeisler CA, Rajaratnam SM, Howard ME. Mental health, substance use, and suicidal ideation among unpaid caregivers of adults in the United States during the COVID-19 pandemic: Relationships to age, race/ethnicity, employment, and caregiver intensity. J Affect Disord. 2021 Dec 1;295:1259-1268. doi:10.1016/j.jad.2021.08.130.

Epub 2021 Sep 3. PMID: 34706440; PMCID: PMC8413485.https://pubmed. ncbi.nlm.nih.gov/34706440/

The Importance of a Good Nights Sleep: 10 Tips for Caregivers. (n.d.). https:// www.seniorlink.com/blog/the-importance-of-a-good-nights-sleep-10-tips-for-caregivers

Lee, M. (2022, August 2). *7 Signs It's Time for Memory Care.* © 2007-2022 AgingCare All Rights Reserved. https://www.agingcare.com/articles/ when-is-it-time-to-place-a-loved-one-with-dementia-188309.htm

Cost of Long Term Care by State | Cost of Care Report | Genworth. (n.d.). https:// www.genworth.com/aging-and-you/finances/cost-of-care.html

Science Daily. (2008). Eating Fish May Prevent Memory Loss And Stroke In Old Age. ScienceDaily. https://www.sciencedaily.com/releases/2008/08/ 080804165312.htm#:~:text=The%20study%20found%20that%20people

An, Y., Feng, L., Zhang, X., Wang, Y., Wang, Y., Tao, L., Qin, Z., & Xiao, R. (2019). Dietary intakes and biomarker patterns of folate, vitamin B6, and vitamin B12 can be associated with cognitive impairment by hypermethylation of redox-related genes NUDT15 and TXNRD1. Clinical Epigenetics, 11(1). https://doi.org/10.1186/s13148-019-0741-y

Krikorian, R., Shidler, M. D., Nash, T. A., Kalt, W., Vinqvist-Tymchuk, M. R., Shukitt-Hale, B., & Joseph, J. A. (2010). Blueberry Supplementation Improves Memory in Older Adults †. Journal of Agricultural and Food Chemistry, 58(7), 3996–4000. https://doi.org/10.1021/jf9029332

National Institute on Aging. (2019, November 30). What Do We Know About Diet and Prevention of Alzheimer's Disease? National Institutes of Health. https://www.nia.nih.gov/health/what-do-we-know-about-diet-and-prevention-alzheimers-disease

Raman, R. (2021, March 31). Ask Our Nutritionist: How Many Calories Does a Healthy 65-year-old Woman Need? Healthline. https://www.healthline. com/nutrition/calories-for-a-healthy-65-year-old-woman#2

Rowe, M. A., Kelly, A., Horne, C., Lane, S., Campbell, J., Lehman, B., Phipps, C., Keller, M., & Benito, A. P. (2009). Reducing dangerous nighttime events in persons with dementia by using a nighttime monitoring system. Alzheimer's & Dementia, 5(5), 419–426. https://doi.org/10.1016/j.jalz.2008.08.005

Bhandari, T. (2021, September 16). Time until dementia symptoms appear can be estimated via brain scan. Washington University School of Medicine in St. Louis. https://medicine.wustl.edu/news/time-until-ddementia-symptoms-appear-can-be-estimated-via-brain-scan/

Team, L. (2021, May 11). Why does dementia cause hallucinations? Lifted. https://www.liftedcare.com/why-does-dementia-cause-hallucinations/

Aalten, P., de Vugt, M. E., Jaspers, N., Jolles, J., & Verhey, F. R. J. (2005). The course of neuropsychiatric symptoms in dementia. Part I:findings from the two-year longitudinal Maasbed study. International Journal of Geriatric Psychiatry, 20(6), 523–530. https://doi.org/10.1002/gps.1316

Prado-Jean, A., Couratier, P., Druet-Cabanac, M., Nubukpo, P., Bernard-Bourzeix, L., Thomas, P., Dechamps, N., Videaud, H., Dantoine, T., & Clément, J. P. (2010). Specific psychological and behavioral symptoms of depression in patients with dementia. International Journal of Geriatric Psychiatry, 25(10), 1065–1072. https://doi.org/10.1002/gps.2468

Savva, G. M., Zaccai, J., Matthews, F. E., Davidson, J. E., McKeith, I., & Brayne, C. (2009). Prevalence, correlates and course of behavioral and psychological symptoms of dementia in the population. British Journal of Psychiatry, 194(3), 212–219. https://doi.org/10.1192/bjp.bp.108.049619

Cerejeira, J., Lagarto, L., & Mukaetova-Ladinska, E. B. (2012). Behavioral and Psychological Symptoms of Dementia. Frontiers in Neurology, 3(73). https://doi.org/10.3389/fneur.2012.00073

Chaudhury, S., & Kiran, C. (2009). Understanding delusions. Industrial Psychiatry Journal, 18(1), 3. https://doi.org/10.4103/0972-6748.57851

Wilson, R. S., Barral, S., Lee, J. H., Leurgans, S. E., Foroud, T. M., Sweet, R. A., Graff-Radford, N., Bird, T. D., Mayeux, R., & Bennett, D. A. (2011). Heritability of Different Forms of Memory in the Late Onset Alzheimer's Disease Family Study. Journal of Alzheimer's Disease, 23(2), 249–255. https://doi.org/10.3233/jad-2010-101515

Sadigh-Eteghad, S., Talebi, M., & Farhoudi, M. (2012). Association of apolipoprotein E epsilon 4 allele with sporadic late onset Alzheimer's disease. Neurosciences, 17(4), 321-326.

Tanaka, M., Török, N., & Vécsei, L. (2021). Novel Pharmaceutical Approaches in Dementia. NeuroPsychopharmacotherapy, 1–18. https://doi.org/10.1007/978-3-319-56015-1_444-1

Noufi, P., Khoury, R., Jeyakumar, S., & Grossberg, G. T. (2019). Use of

Cholinesterase Inhibitors in Non-Alzheimer's Dementias. *Drugs & Aging, 36*(8), 719–731. https://doi.org/10.1007/s40266-019-00685-6

de Vugt, M. E., & Verhey, F. R. J. (2013). The impact of early dementia diagnosis and intervention on informal caregivers. *Progress in Neurobiology, 110,* 54–62. https://doi.org/10.1016/j.pneurobio.2013.04.005

Rasmussen, J., & Langerman, H. (2019). Alzheimer's Disease – Why We Need Early Diagnosis. *Degenerative Neurological and Neuromuscular Disease, Volume 9,* 123–130. https://doi.org/10.2147/dnnd.s228939

Huang, J. (2022). *Delirium - Neurologic Disorders*. MSD Manual Professional Edition. https://www.msdmanuals.com/professional/neurologic-disorders/delirium-and-dementia/delirium

Alzheimer's Association. (2021). *Facts and Figures*. Alzheimer's Disease and Dementia. https://www.alz.org/alzheimers-dementia/facts-figures

Senior Helpers National. (2013). *What is Dementia?* Www.youtube.com. https://www.youtube.com/watch?v=t--mkzfHulE&t=530s

World Health Organization. (2021, September 2). *Dementia*. World Health Organization; World Health Organization: WHO. https://www.who.int/news-room/fact-sheets/detail/dementia

Verma, M., & Howard, R. J. (2012). Semantic memory and language dysfunction in early Alzheimer's disease: a review. *International journal of geriatric psychiatry, 27*(12), 1209–1217. https://doi.org/10.1002/gps.3766

Heron, M. (2021). National vital statistics reports. *National vital statistics reports, 70*(3).

Hugo, J., & Ganguli, M. (2014). Dementia and Cognitive Impairment: Epidemiology, Diagnosis, and Treatment. *Clinics in geriatric medicine, 30*(3), 421. https://doi.org/10.1016/j.cger.2014.04.001

Esposito, L. (2019). *Normal Brain vs. Brain With Dementia*. US News & World Report; U.S. News & World Report. https://health.usnews.com/conditions/brain-disease/dementia/articles/normal-brain-vs-dementia-brain

CDC. (2021, April 7). *What Is Alzheimer's Disease? | CDC*. Www.cdc.gov. https://www.cdc.gov/aging/aginginfo/alzheimers.htm i

Marra, C., Piccininni, C., Masone Iacobucci, G., Caprara, A., Gainotti, G., Costantini, E. M., Callea, A., Venneri, A., & Quaranta, D. (2021). Semantic Memory as an Early Cognitive Marker of Alzheimer's Disease: Role of Category and Phonological Verbal Fluency Tasks. *Journal of Alzheimer's Disease, 81*(2), 619–627. https://doi.org/10.3233/jad-201452

Wolters, F. J., & Ikram, M. A. (2019). Epidemiology of Vascular Dementia. *Arteriosclerosis, Thrombosis, and Vascular Biology, 39*(8), 1542–1549. https://doi.org/10.1161/atvbaha.119.311908

Masson, N. (2022). Stepwise decline is an important clinical feature of vascular cognitive impairment. *Www.bmj.com.* https://www.bmj.com/rapid-response/2011/11/03/stepwise-decline-important-clinical-feature-vascular-cognitive-impairment

Fernandes, C. (2010, November 12). *Diagnosis and Prognosis of Those Living With LBD.* Lewy Body Dementia Association. https://www.lbda.org/diagnosis-and-prognosis/

Precision Vaccination. (2022). *Alzheimer's Disease Vaccines.* Www.precisionvaccinations.com. https://www.precisionvaccinations.com/vaccines/alzheimers-disease-vaccines

Leroy, M., Bertoux, M., Skrobala, E., Mode, E., Adnet-Bonte, C., Le Ber, I., Bombois, S., Cassagnaud, P., Chen, Y., Deramecourt, V., Lebert, F., Mackowiak, M. A., Sillaire, A. R., Wathelet, M., Pasquier, F., & Lebouvier, T. (2021). Characteristics and progression of patients with frontotemporal dementia in a regional memory clinic network. *Alzheimer's Research & Therapy, 13*(1). https://doi.org/10.1186/s13195-020-00753-9

Mild cognitive impairment - Symptoms and causes. (2020, September 2). Mayo Clinic. https://www.mayoclinic.org/diseases-conditions/mild-cognitive-impairment/symptoms-causes/syc-20354578

Parkinson's Foundation. (2019, June 13). *Statistics.* Parkinson's Foundation. https://www.parkinson.org/Understanding-Parkinsons/Statistics

Parkinson, J. (1969). AN ESSAY ON THE SHAKING PALSY. *Archives of Neurology, 20*(4), 441–445. https://doi.org/10.1001/archneur.1969.00480100117017

Satery, J. (2020, February 14). *5 Foods Older Adults with Dementia Should Avoid.* Home Care Assistance of Arlington. https://www.homecareassistancearlingtontx.com/foods-for-elderly-people-to-avoid-if-they-have-dementia/

Boston University Arts & Sciences. (n.d.). Retrieved November 6, 2022, from https://www.bu.edu/cas/magazine/spring10/golomb/

Baugh, C. M., Robbins, C. A., Stern, R. A., & McKee, A. C. (2014). Current Understanding of Chronic Traumatic Encephalopathy. *Current Treatment Options in Neurology, 16*(9). https://doi.org/10.1007/s11940-014-0306-5

Breen, P. W., & Krishnan, V. (2020). Recent Preclinical Insights Into the

Treatment of Chronic Traumatic Encephalopathy. *Frontiers in Neuroscience, 14.* https://doi.org/10.3389/fnins.2020.00616

Zlokovic, B. V. (2011). Neurovascular pathways to neurodegeneration in Alzheimer's disease and other disorders. *Nature Reviews Neuroscience, 12*(12), 723–738. https://doi.org/10.1038/nrn3114

Cui, K., Song, R., Xu, H., Shang, Y., Qi, X., Buchman, A. S., Bennett, D. A., & Xu, W. (2020). Association of Cardiovascular Risk Burden With Risk and Progression of Disability: Mediating Role of Cardiovascular Disease and Cognitive Decline. *Journal of the American Heart Association, 9*(18). https://doi.org/10.1161/jaha.120.017346

Camandola, S., & Mattson, M. P. (2017). Brain metabolism in health, aging, and neurodegeneration. *The EMBO Journal, 36*(11), 1474–1492. https://doi.org/10.15252/embj.201695810

Zhang, J. (2019). Basic Neural Units of the Brain: Neurons, Synapses and Action Potential. *ArXiv:1906.01703 [Q-Bio].* https://arxiv.org/abs/1906.01703

Serra, L., D'Amelio, M., Di Domenico, C., Dipasquale, O., Marra, C., Mercuri, N. B., Caltagirone, C., Cercignani, M., & Bozzali, M. (2018). In vivo mapping of brainstem nuclei functional connectivity disruption in Alzheimer's disease. *Neurobiology of Aging, 72,* 72–82. https://doi.org/10.1016/j.neurobiolaging.2018.08.012

Lyketsos, C. G., Lopez, O., Jones, B., Fitzpatrick, A. L., Breitner, J., & DeKosky, S. (2002). Prevalence of neuropsychiatric symptoms in dementia and mild cognitive impairment: results from the cardiovascular health study. JAMA, 288(12), 1475–1483. https://doi.org/10.1001/jama.288.12.1475

Image References

Blausen.com staff (2014). "Medical gallery of Blausen Medical 2014".

WikiJournal of Medicine 1 (2). DOI:10.15347/wjm/2014.010. ISSN 2002-4436

Young, KA., Wise, JA., DeSaix, P., Kruse, DH., Poe, B., Johnson, E., Johnson, JE., Korol, O., Betts, JG., & Womble, M., CC BY 4.0< https://creativecommons.org/licenses/by/4.0>, via Wikimedia Commons. https://upload.wikimedia.org/wikipedia/commons/3/37/1225_Chemical_Synapse.jpg

File:Blausen 0111 BrainLobes.png - Wikimedia Commons. (2014, February 11).

https://commons.wikimedia.org/wiki/File:
Blausen_0111_BrainLobes.png

BruceBlaus, CC BY-SA 4.0 <https://creativecommons.org/licenses/by-sa/4.0>,via Wikimedia Commons. https://upload.wikimedia.org/wiki pedia/commons/9/99/Alzheimers_Disease.jpg

Triff. (n.d.). Closeup of a CT scan with brain. Medical, science and education mri brain background. [Online Image]. In Shutterstock. Retrieved September 25,

Kon, K. (n.d.). 3D illustration showing neurons containing Lewy bodies [Online Image]. In Shutterstock. Retrieved September 26, 2022, from https://www.shutterstock.com/image-illustration/parkinsons-disease-3d-illustration-showing-neurons-746439844

lukpedclub. (n.d.). pain measurement scale, line icon with fill color for assessment tool [Online Image]. In Shutterstock. Retrieved October 4, 2022, from https://www.shutterstock.com/image-vector/pain-measurement-scale-line-icon-fill-693213469

File:Suprachiasmatic Nucleus.jpg - Wikimedia Commons. (2014, January 7). https://commons.wikimedia.org/wiki/File:Suprachiasmatic_Nucleus.jpg https://commons.wikimedia.org/wiki/File:Suprachiasmatic_Nucleus.jpg